Bedside Ultrasound

Level 1

PETER STEINMETZ, MD

First Edition-Revised

Consultant Editors:

André Denault, MD, PhD, ABIM-CCM, FASE, FRCPC

David McAuley, MD, FRCP-C, ABR

Philippe Rola, MD, FRCP-C

Includes online instructional videos:
bedsideultrasoundlevel1.com

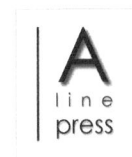

A
line
press

First Edition

first printing, June 2013

second printing, October 2013

third printing, February 2014; Revisions include new figures (Figures 3.6, 7.6, 10.2), new figures in the 'Case closed' section of each chapter, expanded Summary (page 78), and correction of minor typographical errors.

Library and Archives Canada Cataloguing in Publication

Steinmetz, Peter, 1963-, author

Bedside ultrasound / Peter Steinmetz, MD ; consultant editors: André Denault, MD, PhD, ABIM-CCM, FASE, FRCPC; David McAuley, MD, FRCP-C, ABR; Philippe Rola, MD, FRCP-C. -- Level 1.

"Includes online instructional videos: bedsideultrasoundlevel1.com".

Illustrator: Dr Sharon Oleskevich, PhD.

Includes bibliographical references and index.

ISBN 978-0-9919566-0-9 (pbk.)

1. Diagnostic ultrasonic imaging. 2. Point-of-care testing.
I. Oleskevich, Sharon, 1964-, illustrator II. Denault, André, editor   III. Rola, Philippe, 1970-, editor IV. McAuley, David, 1964-, editor V. Title.

RC78.7.U4S74 2013   616.07'543   C2013-902570-7

The information in this book is designed to provide helpful information on the subjects discussed. While best efforts have been made to provide accurate information that is in accord with current standards of practice, the author, editor, or publisher make no warranty with respect to the accuracy or completeness of the contents. Application of the information in a particular situation remains the professional responsibility of the physician. Any likeness to actual persons in the case studies is strictly coincidental. References are provided for informational purposes only and do not constitute endorsement of websites or other sources.

Editing, interior layout, typography
A-line Press

Cover, illustrations, photography
Sharon Oleskevich, PhD

Proofreading
Mark Farso, PhD
Christiane de Brentani, BA

Web design for online videos
John Clements, PhD

Printed and bound in Canada
by Marquis

Published in Canada
by A-line Press

About the Author:

Dr. Peter Steinmetz (MD) works in the intensive care unit at St. Mary's Hospital in Montreal and is Faculty Lecturer in the Department of Family Medicine at McGill University, Canada. He is Director and founder of the Undergraduate Bedside Ultrasound Course at McGill University, and Director of postgraduate and CME courses at the Arnold and Blema Steinberg Medical Simulation Centre. He has taught bedside ultrasound in North America, Asia, and Africa.

About the Consultant Editors:

Dr. André Denault (MD, PhD, ABIM-CCM, FASE, FRCPC) is a cardiac anesthetist at the Institut de Cardiologie de Montréal, and an intensivist at the Centre Hospitalier de l'Université de Montréal. He learned echocardiography as an internist at McGill University. He has authored two textbooks in transesophageal echocardiography and numerous publications in bedside echocardiography. Dr. Denault has been involved in training and teaching bedside echocardiography since 1997 at the Université de Montréal and worldwide.

Dr. David McAuley (MD, FRCP-C, ABR) is Chief of the Department of Radiology at the Centre de Santé du Sud Ouest Verdun, in Montreal. He completed a residency in family medicine at McGill University and went on to certify in emergency medicine (CCFP-EM). He worked as an emergency physician before completing a residency in radiology at McGill University. His fellowship training was in abdominal imaging and non-vascular intervention.

Dr. Philippe Rola (MD, FRCP-C) is an internist trained at McGill University. Dr. Rola is the Director of Intensive Care, Santa Cabrini Hospital in Montreal and works in the intensive care unit at Scarborough General Hospital, Toronto. As founder of the Critical Care Ultrasound Institute, he teaches bedside ultrasound at the international level.

Acknowledgements

There are countless people who deserve mention and a word of thanks. They include collaborators and friends who provided feedback on the text. A special nod to those who encouraged the development of undergraduate bedside ultrasound teaching at McGill University, including the McGill University Bedside Ultrasound Interest Group, Donald Boudreau, and Robert Primavesi. Many ultrasound images used in the book are contributions made by colleagues. Hats off to Vicki Noble, Karen Cosby, Daniel Lichtenstein, André Denault, John Lewis, Hugo Villadeval, Hoa Nguyen, Anne Patricia Prevost, Jean-François Lanctot, Maxime Valois, Eric Tremblay, and CCUS.

A special thanks to Sharon Oleskevich for countless hours of design, layout, organization, writing, and general good advice.

P.S.

Contents

Preface

This introductory handbook is a practical reference for healthcare workers starting to apply bedside ultrasound in their daily practice. It aims to articulate the practical and cognitive skills necessary to effectively use this tool.

Clear and simple diagrams as well as digital online ultrasound videos help illustrate concepts outlined in the text.

The digital online ultrasound videos can be accessed at:

bedsideultrasoundlevel1.com

1. Ultrasound basics

1.1. What is ultrasound?

It is useful to understand some basic concepts about ultrasound in order to correctly interpret the images generated by the bedside ultrasound machine.

Ultrasound is a sound wave that oscillates with a frequency greater than 20000 Hz (20000 cycles per second or 20 kHz). The human ear can detect sound waves with frequencies between 0.02-20 kHz. Sound waves above 20 kHz, such as those generated by dog whistles, bat calls, and ultrasound machines, cannot be interpreted as sound by the human ear. These high frequency sound waves are called **ultrasound**.

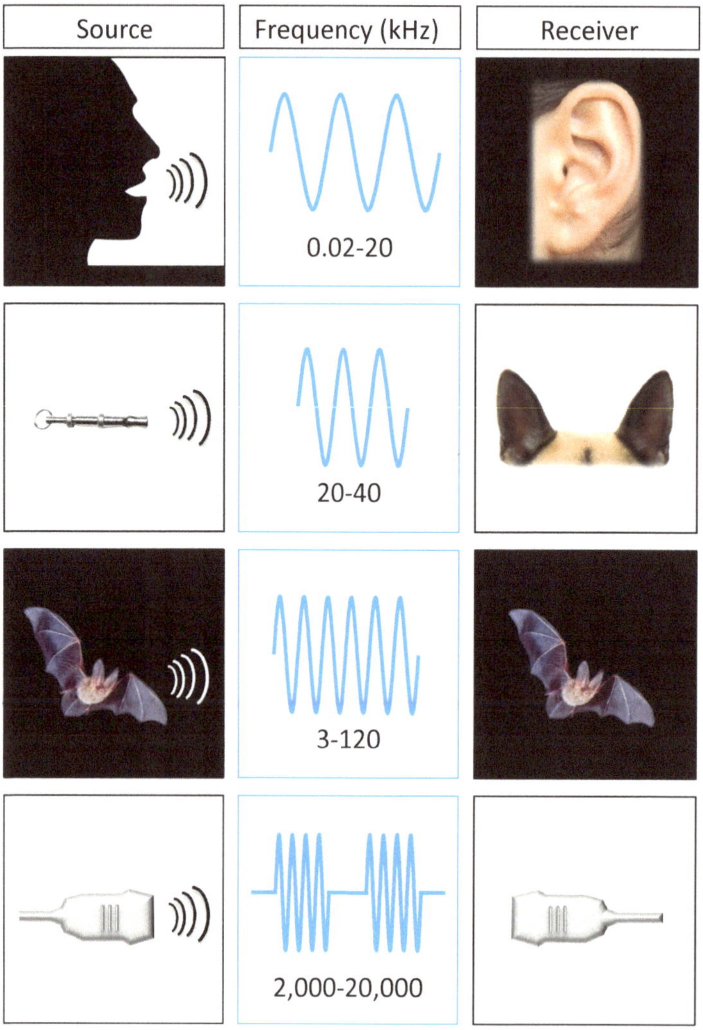

Source	Frequency (kHz)	Receiver
	0.02-20	
	20-40	
	3-120	
	2,000-20,000	

Figure 1.1 Different sound waves and and their frequencies.

The human ear can interpret sound waves with frequencies up to 20 kHz. Sound waves with frequencies above 20 kHz are termed ultrasound. Diagnostic ultrasound ranges in frequency from 2,000-20,000 kHz (2-20 MHz).

1.2. Ultrasound probes send and receive ultrasound

Ultrasound probes have two functions: to send and receive ultrasound. An ultrasound probe spends 1% of its time sending and 99% of its time receiving sound waves.

The probe starts by sending out bursts of ultrasound. When ultrasound encounters a structure, it reflects off that structure and returns to the probe as an echo. The returning echoes are interpreted and expressed as an image on the ultrasound machine monitor.

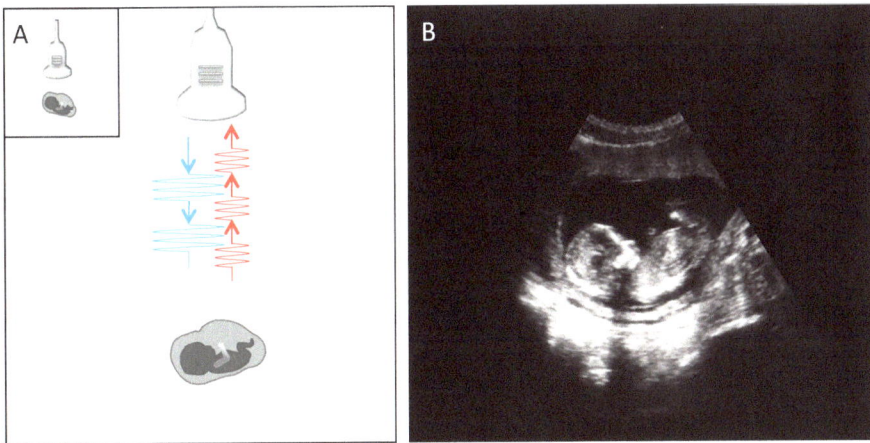

Figure 1.2 Ultrasound probes send and receive ultrasound.

A. Schematic demonstrating a probe sending out sound waves (blue) that encounter tissues and are reflected back as echoes (red).
B. The echoes are detected by the same probe and translated into an ultrasound image.

1.3. How does ultrasound behave travelling through tissue?

Attenuation

Attenuation describes the dampening of the amplitude of ultrasound as it travels through tissue. Attenuation occurs as ultrasound energy is converted into heat, absorbed by a structure, reflected back to the probe, or scattered away from the probe.

Attenuation is directly proportional to the distance that the ultrasound travels and to the ultrasound wavelength. Attenuation is also affected by the characteristics of the medium encountered.

Distance: Attenuation of ultrasound increases as the ultrasound propagates deeper into the body. When imaging the abdomen, the far-field (deeper) structures can appear darker due to attenuation of the ultrasound.

Wavelength: High frequency ultrasound attenuates more rapidly than low frequency ultrasound. Thus, high frequency probes cannot be used to image deep structures.

Type of medium: Air and bone cause a high degree of attenuation. Fluid causes a low degree of attenuation.

Reflection

An image is generated by the ultrasound waves that are reflected from a structure and returned to the probe. The image appears brighter as the amount of reflection increases. In general, reflection is greatest when ultrasound encounters a structure of high-density or when it crosses an interface between structures of different densities.

Hyperechoic: Bone appears hyperechoic (**white**) on the ultrasound image. Its high-density and the interface between surrounding structures of lower density cause a high degree of reflection.

Hypoechoic: Muscle and liver appear hypoechoic (**grey**) on the ultrasound image due to their moderate density.

Anechoic: Fluid (blood, ascites, pleural effusions) appears anechoic (**black**) on the ultrasound image. This is because ultrasound travels through low-density structures with minimal attenuation and reflection back to the ultrasound probe.

Table 1.1 Ultrasound image terminology.

Medium	Terminology	Appearance on ultrasound image	Density of structure
Bone	Hyperechoic	White	High
Muscle, liver	Hypoechoic	Grey	Moderate
Fluid	Anechoic	Black	Low

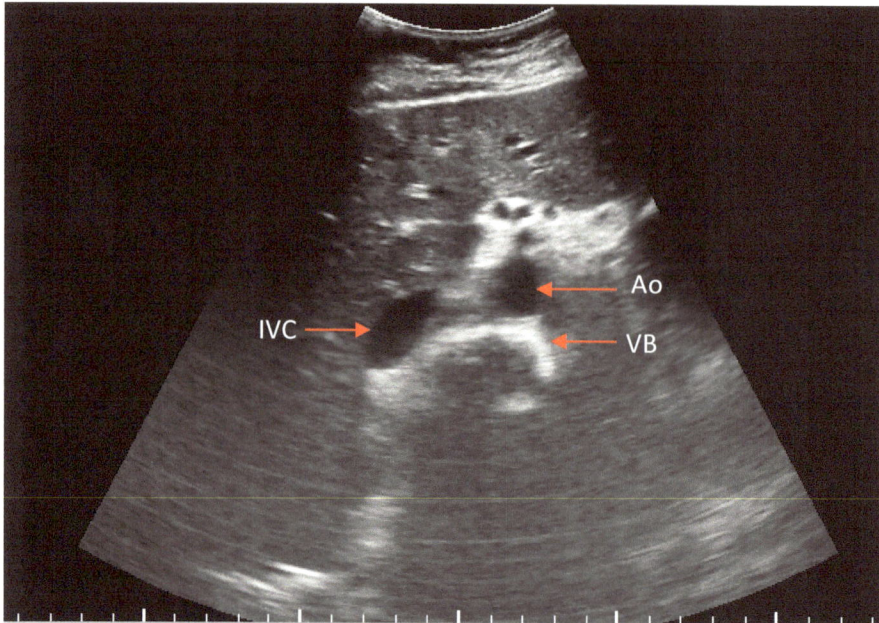

Figure 1.3 Appearance of structures with different densities.

The vertebral body (VB) is a bony, high-density structure that appears hyperechoic (white) on the ultrasound image. The aorta (Ao) and inferior vena cava (IVC) are low-density structures that appear anechoic (black). The tissues surrounding these structures are of moderate density and so appear hypoechoic (varying shades of grey).

1.4. Gain

Due to the attenuation of the ultrasound returning to the probe, structures may appear dark and hard to identify on the image. Increasing the gain on the ultrasound machine increases the signal amplification of the returning attenuated ultrasound. This adjustment makes structures appear hyperechoic (white) on the screen and easier to identify.

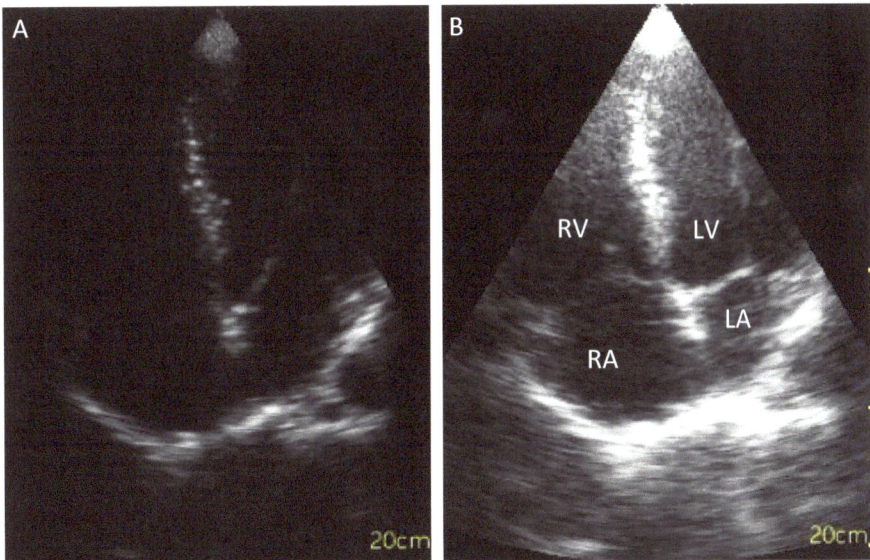

Figure 1.4 Gain adjustment.

A. Ultrasound image showing an apical four chamber view of the heart. With low gain, structures appear dark on the screen.
B. Same image with high gain, structures now appear brighter on the screen.
LV: left ventricle, LA: left atrium, RA: right atrium, RV: right ventricle.

1.5. Depth

Ultrasound machines determine the depth of a structure by measuring the time it takes for a waveform to leave the probe, reflect off the structure, and then return to the probe.

Ultrasound striking superficial structures will return to the probe first, followed by ultrasound returning after striking deeper structures. For example, if you are performing an ultrasound of the abdomen on a supine patient, the aorta lies superficial to the vertebral bodies. Therefore an ultrasound waveform leaving the probe will reflect off the aorta and return to the probe before it reflects off the vertebral body and returns to the probe. The ultrasound machine interprets this time difference and generates an image with the aorta superficial to the vertebral body.

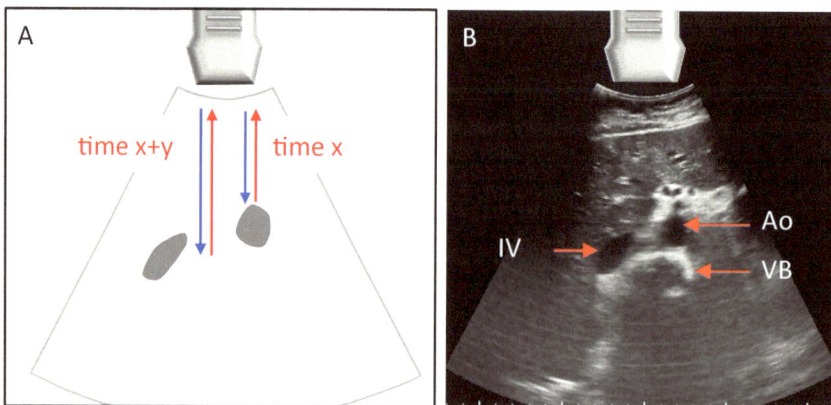

Figure 1.5 Ultrasound machines determine the depth of a structure.
A. *The depth of the structure determines the time for ultrasound to travel from the probe to the structure and back again. The round-trip time is longer for deeper structures.*
B. *Corresponding ultrasound image demonstrating the aorta (Ao) superficial to the vertebral body (VB). IVC: inferior vena cava.*

The depth of the ultrasound field can be adjusted by changing how often the signal is emitted from the probe. Adjust the depth setting on the ultrasound machine such that structures of interest can be viewed in the middle of the ultrasound field.

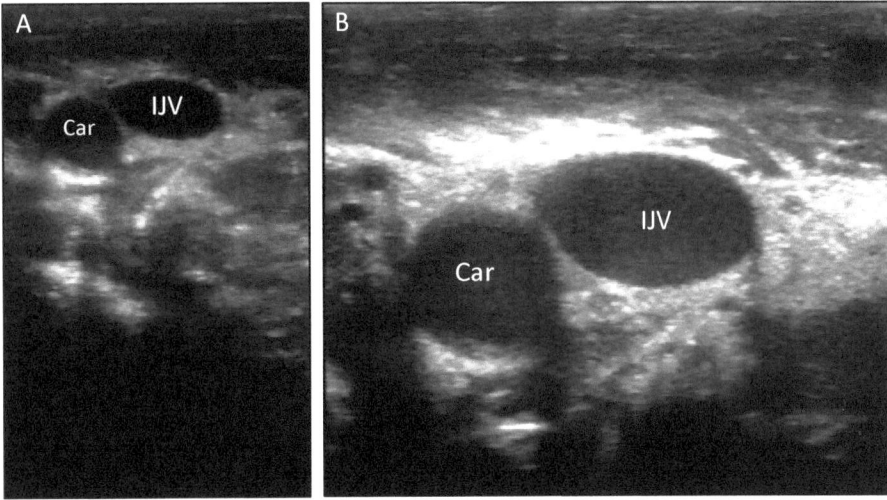

Figure 1.6 Depth adjustment.

A. Depth setting is too high. The internal jugular vein (IJV) is too high in the field of view and difficult to identify.
B. Lower depth setting. Same vessels in the middle of the field appear larger and easier to identify. Car: carotid artery.

1.6. Ultrasound frequency dictates resolution and depth

The choice of ultrasound probe depends on the required resolution and the depth of the structure to be imaged because of the following two principles:

Principle #1: The frequency of the ultrasound wavelength is proportional to the degree of resolution. Thus, low frequency sound waves provide low resolution while high frequency sound waves provide high resolution.

Principle #2: The frequency of the ultrasound wavelength is inversely proportional to the degree of penetration. Thus, low frequency sound waves travel further into the tissue and can image deep structures. High frequency sound waves travel a shorter distance and are used to image superficial structures.

Summary: A low frequency probe is a good choice to produce low resolution images of large deep structures.

A high frequency probe is a good choice to produce high resolution images of small superficial structures.

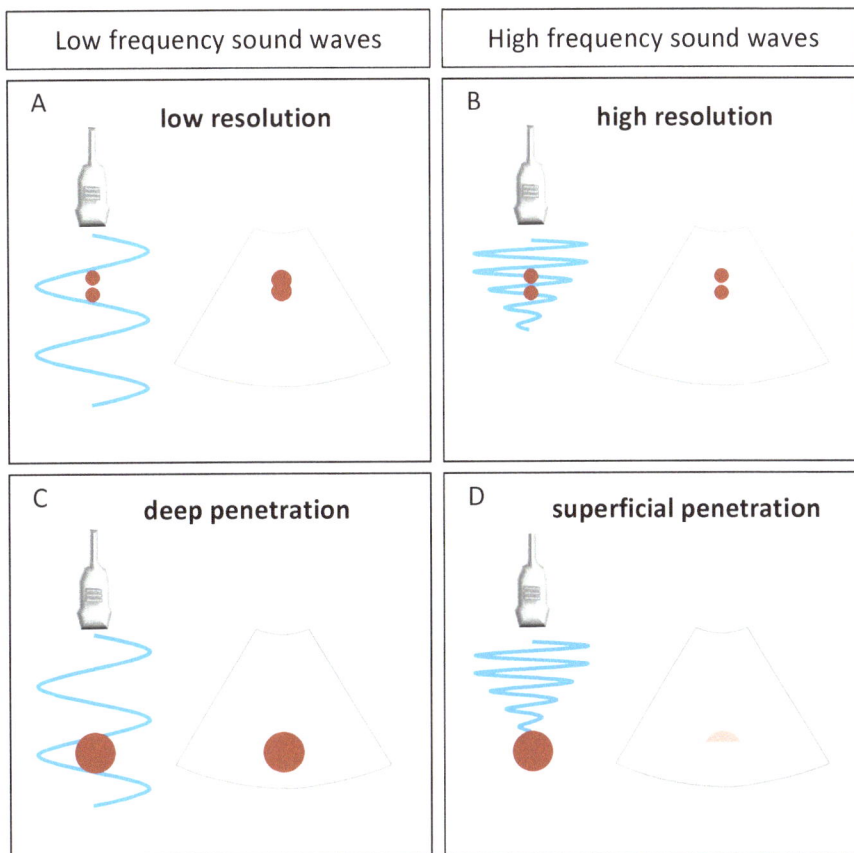

Figure 1.7. Frequency of ultrasound dictates resolution and depth.

A. Low frequency sound waves provide a low resolution ultrasound image.
B. High frequency sound waves provide a high resolution ultrasound image.
C. Low frequency sound waves can image deep structures.
D. High frequency sound waves cannot image deep structures.

1.7. Doppler and flow

As ultrasound is reflected from moving objects like flowing blood, the frequency of the returning waveform is altered. This frequency shift is described by the Doppler principle. The frequency of the reflected ultrasound is increased when blood flow is towards the probe. The frequency of the reflected ultrasound is decreased when blood flow is away from the probe.

The direction of blood flow relative to the probe is represented by different colors on the ultrasound image. One commonly used convention is that flow away from the probe is colored blue and flow towards the probe is colored red. This convention can be remembered using the acronym **BART**.

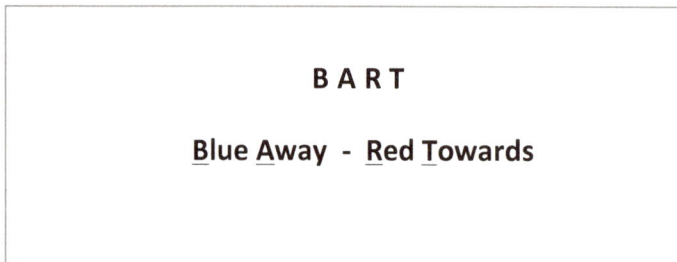

B A R T

Blue Away - Red Towards

The Doppler principle is useful for differentiating arteries from veins. As shown in Figure 1.8, when the ultrasound beam is directed caudally and towards the heart (A-B), flow in the jugular vein is away from the probe (blue) and flow in the carotid artery is towards the probe (red).

Reversing the ultrasound beam by pointing the probe cephalad (C-D) reverses the colored representations because the direction of flow relative to the probe has been reversed.

There is no frequency shift when the ultrasound beam is directed perpendicular to blood flow (E-F) and therefore no colored representation.

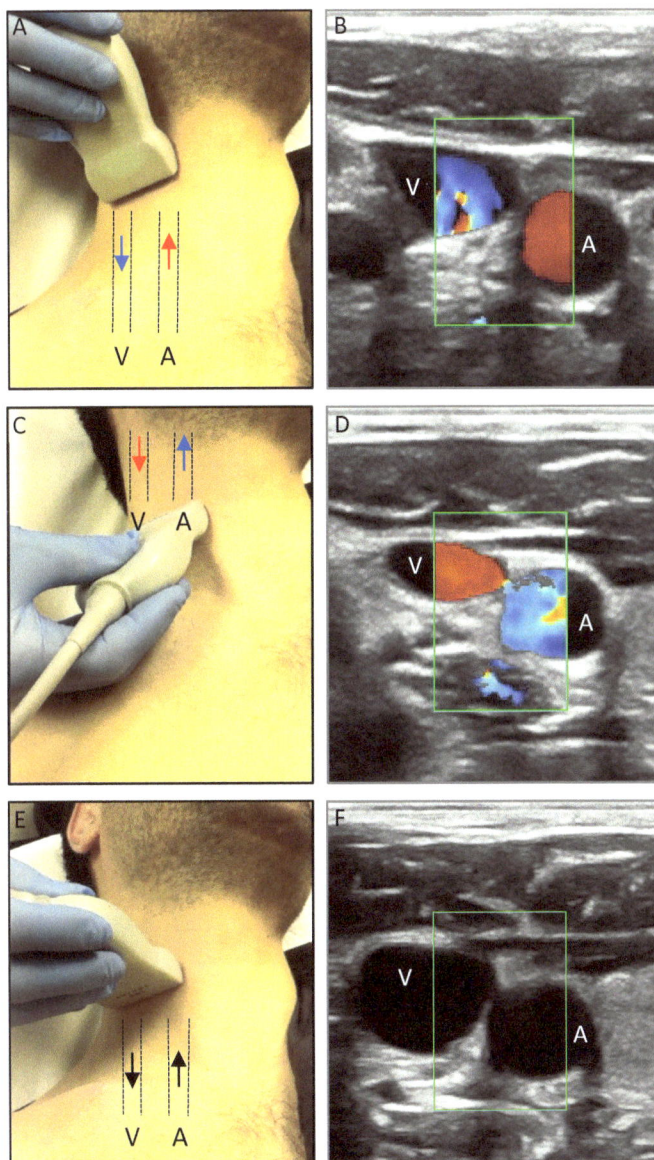

Figure 1.8 Using Doppler and 'BART' to assess direction of blood flow.

A-B. When the probe is pointing caudally, venous flow is away from the probe (blue) and arterial flow is towards the probe (red).
C-D. When the probe is pointing cephalad, venous flow is towards the probe (red) and arterial flow is away from the probe (blue).
E-F. No color is generated when the probe is held perpendicular to flow.
V: Jugular vein, A: Carotid artery.

2. Image generation

2.1. Probe choice

The choice of probe depends on the depth of the structure being imaged. Low frequency probes provide the penetration necessary to image deep structures. High frequency probes provide excellent imaging of small superficial structures.

Table 2.1 Appropriate probe choice for imaging different structures.

Low frequency probe (2-6 MHz)	High frequency probe (5-14 MHz)
Heart	Vessels
Gallbladder	Nerves
Kidney	Pleura
Bladder	Eye
Liver	Soft tissue
Spleen	Testicle

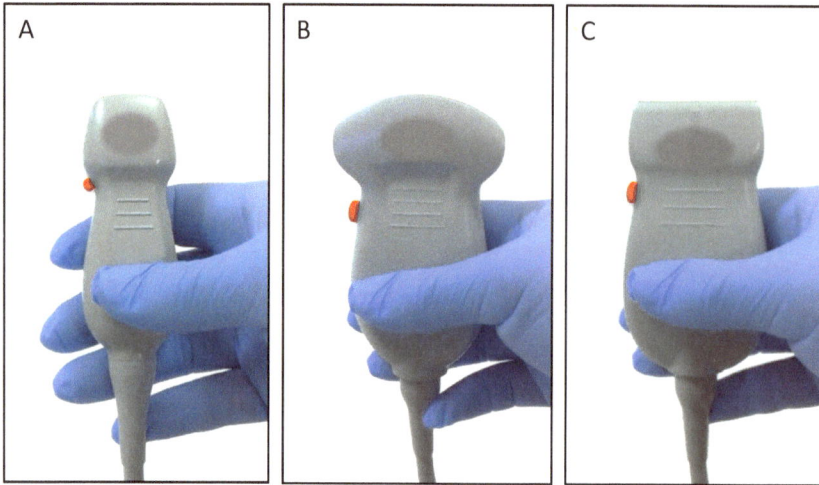

Figure 2.1 Three commonly used probes.

A. The low frequency phased array probe is used for imaging heart, lung, and abdomen.

B. The low frequency curvilinear probe is used for imaging abdominal structures.

C. The high frequency linear probe is used for imaging superficial structures. Red circle denotes orientation marker.

2.2. Sonographer and patient position

The position of both the sonographer and the patient must be optimized to ensure acquisition of high quality images. The height of the patient's bed should be adjusted so that the ultrasonographer is comfortable. Awkward positioning will cause the ultrasonographer to tire and be unable to obtain adequate images. Resting part of the hand on the patient may decrease fatigue, enhance image stability, and enable small, controlled movements.

Due to space and time constraints in bedside ultrasound, the sonographer should learn to obtain images from either side of the patient.

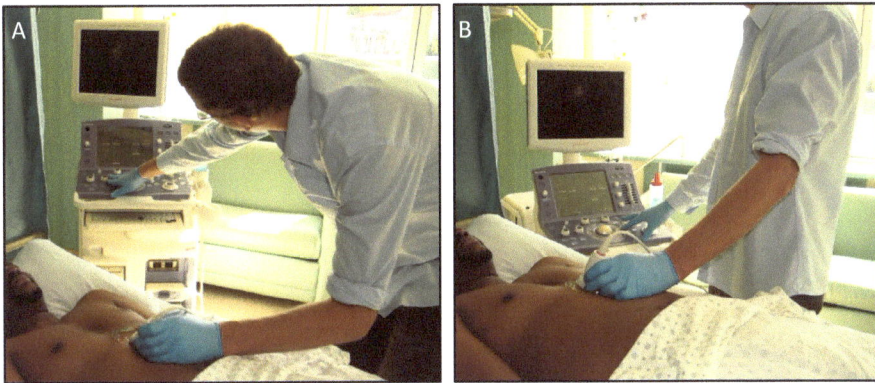

Figure 2.2 Ultrasonographer position.
A. _Incorrect position:_ the bed is too low and the screen is facing away from the sonographer. The ultrasonographer will soon tire and is unlikely to generate adequate images.
B. _Correct position:_ the ultrasonographer is well placed to orient the probe, view the screen, and adjust settings.

There are many examples when the patient's position is important to obtain optimal images.

Table 2.2 Body structure and patient position for optimal ultrasound images.

Structure	Patient position for optimal images
Lung	Supine
Heart - apical four chamber view	Left lateral decubitus
Heart - parasternal long view	Left lateral decubitus
Kidney - left	Supine or right lateral decubitus
Kidney - right	Supine or left lateral decubitus
Gallbladder	Supine or left lateral decubitus
Free abdominal fluid	Supine
Aorta	Supine, or lying on either side for obese patients
Neck veins	Supine
Leg venous study for deep venous thrombosis (DVT)	Supine with head elevated, or sitting for ambulatory patients

2.3. Use enough gel

Ultrasound waves scatter when they encounter air. To avoid air being trapped between the probe surface and the patient's body, gel is applied between the probe surface and the body. The gel allows the ultrasound waves to travel between the probe and the body without scattering.

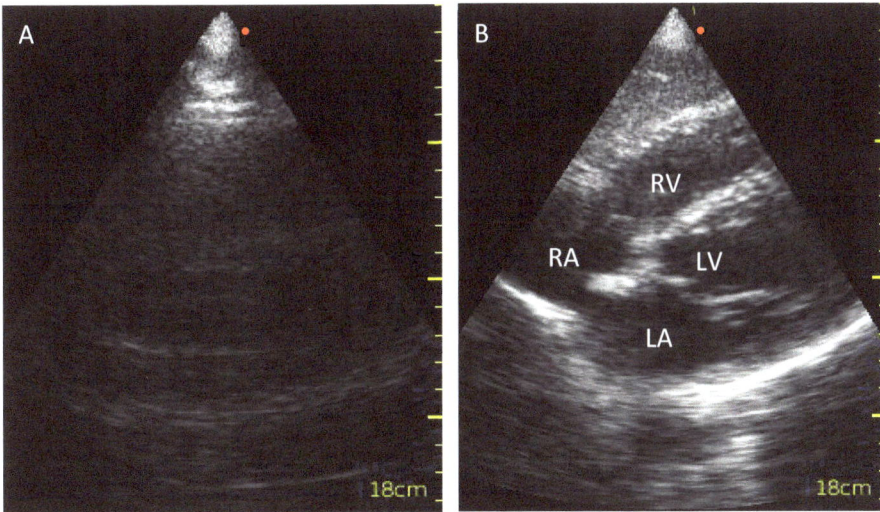

Figure 2.3 Two subxiphoid images of the heart.

A. The image to the left was obtained with insufficient gel, resulting in an artifact obscuring the heart.
B. Same view but with adequate gel applied.
LV: left ventricle, LA: left atrium, RA: right atrium, RV: right ventricle. Red circle denotes orientation marker.

2.4. Identify structure of interest

As the probe makes contact with the patient, slowly scan until the structure of interest appears on the monitor of the ultrasound machine.

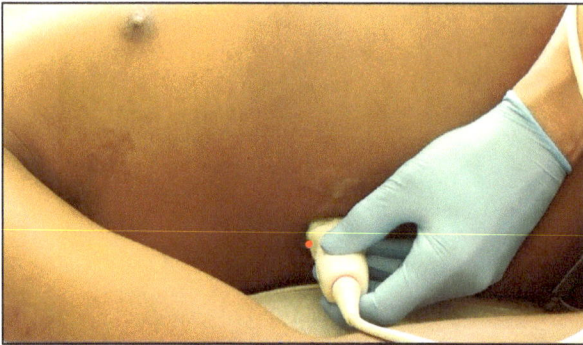

Video 2.1 Scan slowly to identify the structure of interest.

The probe must be moved slowly to identify the right kidney. Red circle denotes orientation marker. View video online at bedsideultrasoundlevel1.com

2.5. Understanding the ultrasound image

The body is divided into sagittal, coronal, and transverse planes.

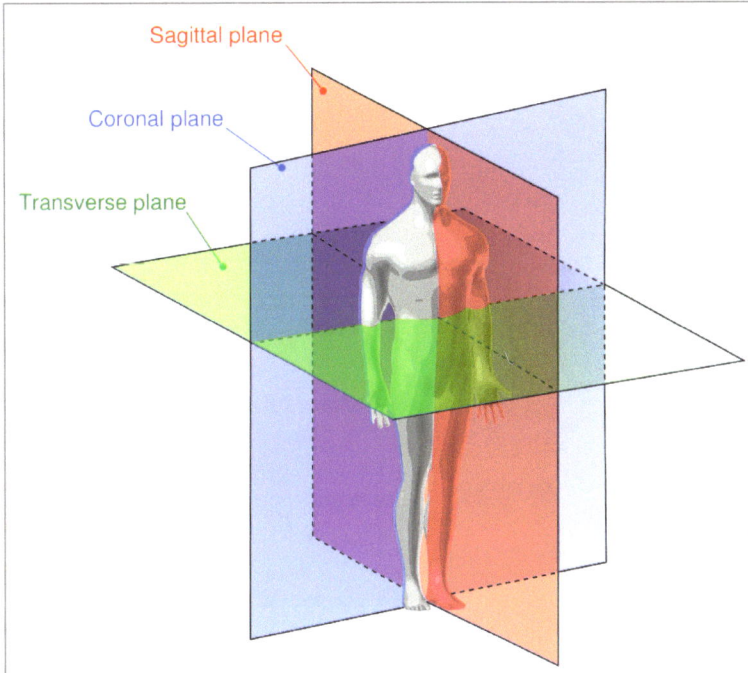

Figure 2.4 The three body planes (Mrabet, 2012).

As the structure of interest appears on the ultrasound machine monitor, the plane of the image is dictated by the orientation of the ultrasound probe.

For example, to obtain an image of the abdomen in the transverse plane, the probe is placed on the anterior abdomen with the orientation marker pointing to the patient's right.

To obtain an image of the abdomen in the sagittal plane, the probe is placed on the anterior abdomen with the orientation marker pointing cephalad.

To obtain an image of the abdomen in the coronal plane, the probe is placed over the lateral abdomen with the orientation marker pointing cephalad.

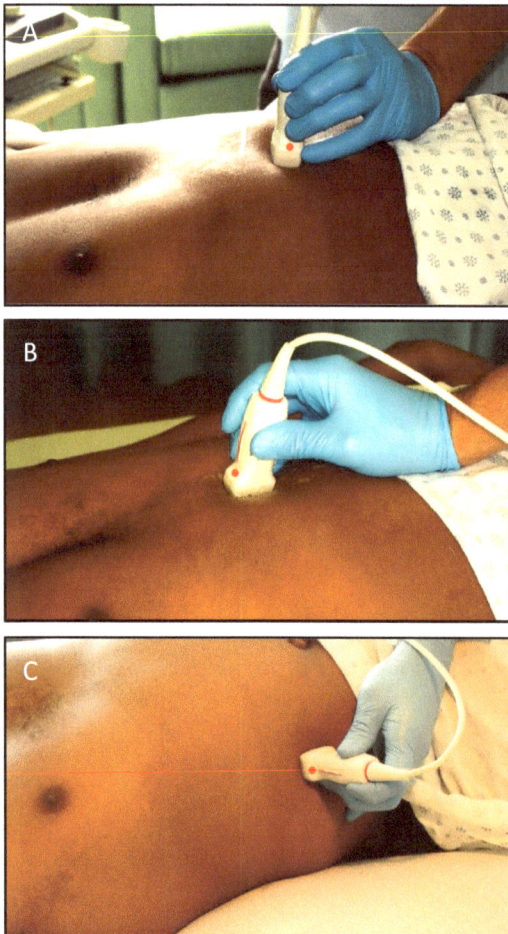

Figure 2.5 Probe placement.
Probe placement for generation of abdominal images in the transverse (A), sagittal (B), and coronal (C) planes. Red circle denotes orientation marker.

Field of view

Ultrasound probes generate different shaped fields of view on the ultrasound monitor. For example, high frequency linear probes generate rectangular fields of view. Low frequency phased array or curvilinear probes generate triangular fields of view.

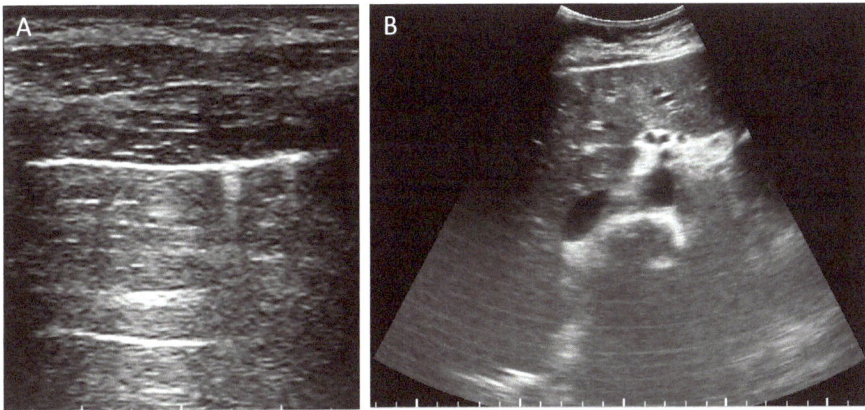

Figure 2.6 Fields of view generated by different probes.
A. Field of view generated by a high frequency linear probe.
B. Field of view generated by a low frequency phased array or curvilinear probe.

The field of view is divided into near-field and far-field. Near-field structures are superficial while far-field structures are deep.

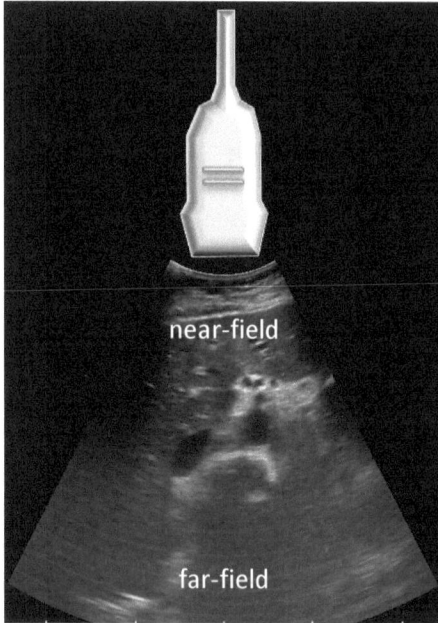

Figure 2.7 The ultrasound image is divided into near-field and far-field.

Orientation of structures relative to probe position

Every probe has an orientation marker located on the side of the probe that corresponds to an orientation marker on the field of view. By noting the alignment of the orientation marker on the probe and the screen, the sonographer can keep track of where structures are situated relative to each other.

'Abdominal setting'

Consider an image of the abdomen in the transverse plane. The image is generated by placing a probe on the abdomen with the orientation marker pointing to the patient's right. The orientation marker will appear on the upper left corner of the screen. This is the convention when probes are used in the 'abdominal setting'. Therefore structures on the patient's right appear on the left of the ultrasound field of view.

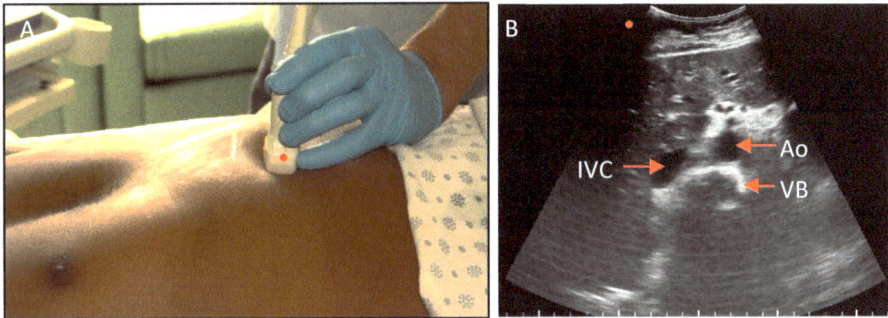

Figure 2.8 Alignment of orientation markers on the probe and ultrasound screen.

A. Imaging abdominal structures in the transverse plane with a phased array probe in the 'abdominal setting'. The orientation marker is to the patient's right.

B. The orientation marker appears on the upper left corner of the screen. The inferior vena cava (IVC) is to the left of the aorta (Ao) on the ultrasound screen. VB: vertebral body. Red circle denotes orientation marker.

'Cardiac setting'

Due to convention, the orientation marker will appear on the upper right hand corner of the screen when imaging the heart with any probe in the 'cardiac setting'.

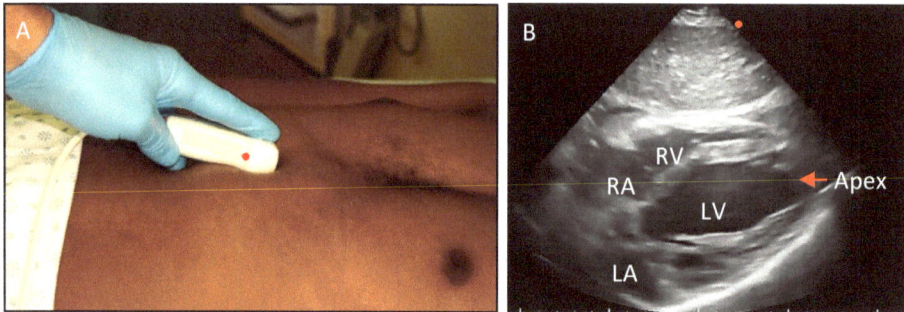

Figure 2.9 Alignment of orientation markers on the probe and ultrasound screen for imaging the heart.

A. Imaging the heart with a phased array probe in the 'cardiac setting'. The orientation marker on the probe is to the patient's left.
B. The orientation marker appears on the upper right corner of the screen. The apex of the heart appears on the right side of the ultrasound screen. LV: left ventricle, LA: left atrium, RA: right atrium, RV: right ventricle. Red circle denotes orientation marker.

2.6. Adjust depth

When the structure of interest appears on the ultrasound screen, adjust the depth such that the structure appears centered in the screen. This adjustment will improve the quality of the image.

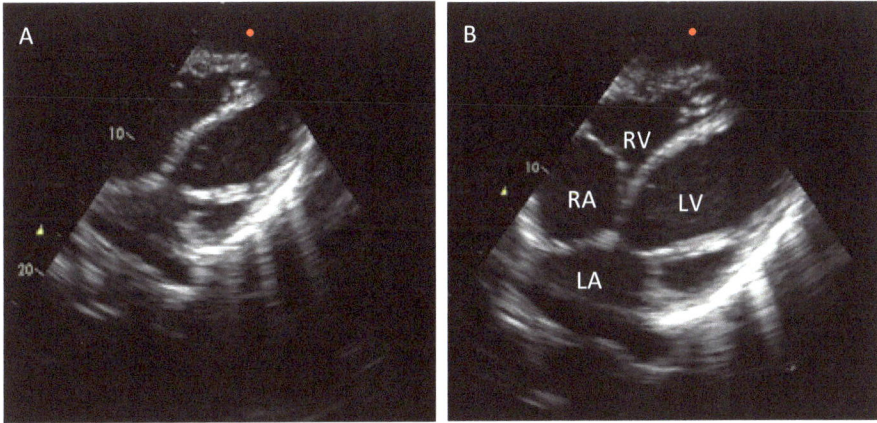

Figure 2.10 Adjusting the depth to improve the quality of the image.
A. Subxiphoid view of the heart with depth setting too deep.
B. Same view with correct depth setting.
LV: left ventricle, LA: left atrium, RA: right atrium, RV: right ventricle. Red circle denotes orientation marker.

2.7. Adjust gain

When gain is set too low, the image will appear dark on the screen. When gain is set too high, the image will appear white on the screen. Adjust the gain to optimize the quality of the image and improve your ability to identify structures of interest.

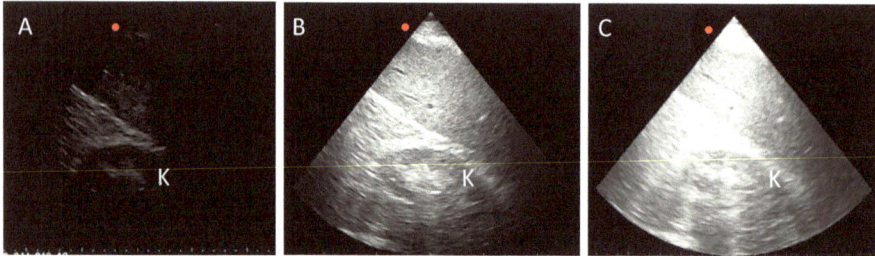

Figure 2.11 Adjusting the gain to optimize the quality of the image.
A. View of the kidney (K) with gain set too low.
B. Same kidney with correct gain setting.
C. Same kidney with gain set too high.
Red circle denotes orientation marker.

2.8. Cleaning the machine and the patient

Since portable ultrasound machines are used on different patients, one must avoid allowing the machines to become vectors for nosocomial disease. Therefore, it is imperative that the ultrasonographer follows the manufacturer's recommendations regarding the proper cleaning of the machine between patients and uses gloves when examining a patient.

2.9. Troubleshooting tips

- To improve image quality, ensure the following are optimal:

  - ➢ patient position

  - ➢ probe choice

  - ➢ gel usage

  - ➢ gain setting

  - ➢ depth setting

- To improve image quality, it is important to orient the probe perpendicular to the structure of interest. This procedure minimizes the scatter of ultrasound and maximizes the quantity of ultrasound reflected back to the probe.

3. Artifacts

3.1. Common artifacts

Artifacts are images that do not represent an anatomic structure. They are generated due to the behavior of ultrasound interacting with structures within the body. It is important to recognize artifacts so that they are not mistaken for true structures within the body.

In this chapter we introduce four common artifacts. Each artifact offers both an advantage and disadvantage to the ultrasonographer.

Four common artifacts

1. **Shadowing artifact**
2. **Enhancement artifact**
3. **Mirror image artifact**
4. **Reverberation artifact**

3.2. Shadowing artifact

When ultrasound encounters high-density structures like bone or gallstones, all of the ultrasound is either absorbed by or reflected away from the surface of the structure. The surface of the structure appears hyperechoic (white). The area deep to bone or gallstones appears anechoic (black) because there is no ultrasound available deep to these structures. We call this black area a "shadow".

Air also causes shadowing. This is because the large difference in density between air and surrounding tissues cause the sound waves to scatter.

Advantage

Artifacts can be used for identifying a structure. For example, both gallbladder polyps and gallstones can appear as similar protrusions from the gallbladder wall. However, only gallstones produce a shadow deep to their image because of their high-density.

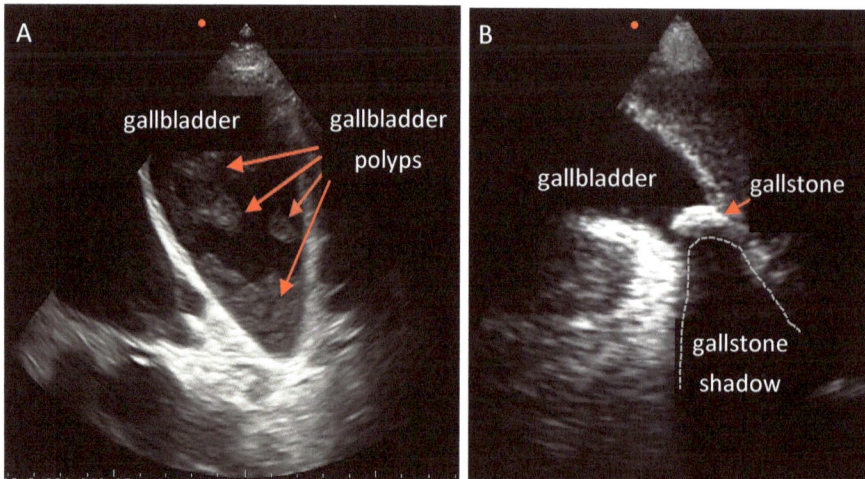

Figure 3.1 Artifacts can be an advantage.
A. An image showing gallbladder polyps. Note that the structures protruding from the gallbladder wall are not producing shadows.
B. This image shows a gallstone, with a characteristic dark shadow deep to the stone. Red circle denotes orientation marker.

Disadvantage

Shadows can be a disadvantage when they obstruct the view of a deeper structure.

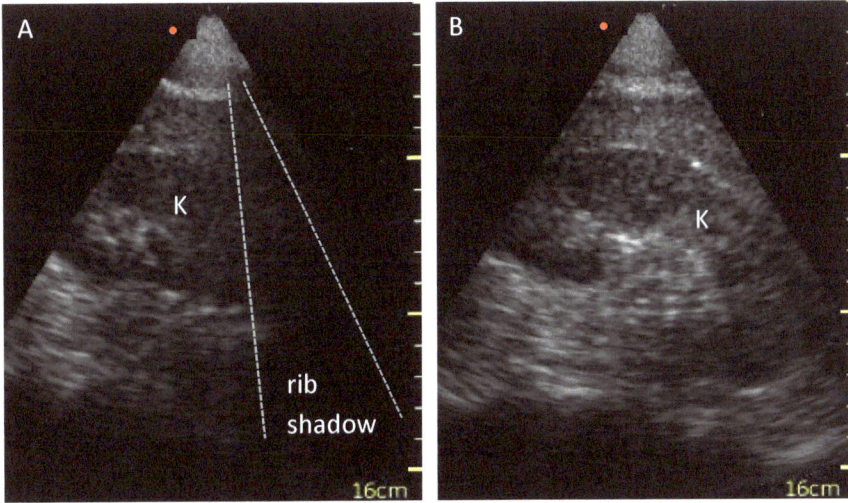

Figure 3.2 Artifacts can be a disadvantage.
A. Ultrasound image of the kidney (K) is obstructed by a rib shadow.
B. The rib shadow is eliminated when the same kidney is viewed from between the ribs. Red circle denotes orientation marker.

3.3. Enhancement artifact

When ultrasound passes through a low-density fluid filled structure, such as a gallbladder or a fluid filled cyst, most of the ultrasound travels through the structure with little attenuation. The ultrasound then reaches the interface between the low-density structure and a deeper structure with higher density. There is a high degree of reflection from this interface back to the ultrasound probe. This effect results in the area deep to low-density structures being "enhanced" and appearing hyperechoic (white).

Advantage

An enhancement artifact can be used to differentiate between a fluid filled cyst and a tumor. Both can appear as circular structures within a solid organ. The fluid filled cyst, with its low density, will produce an enhancement artifact. The tumor, with its higher density, will produce less, if any, enhancement artifact.

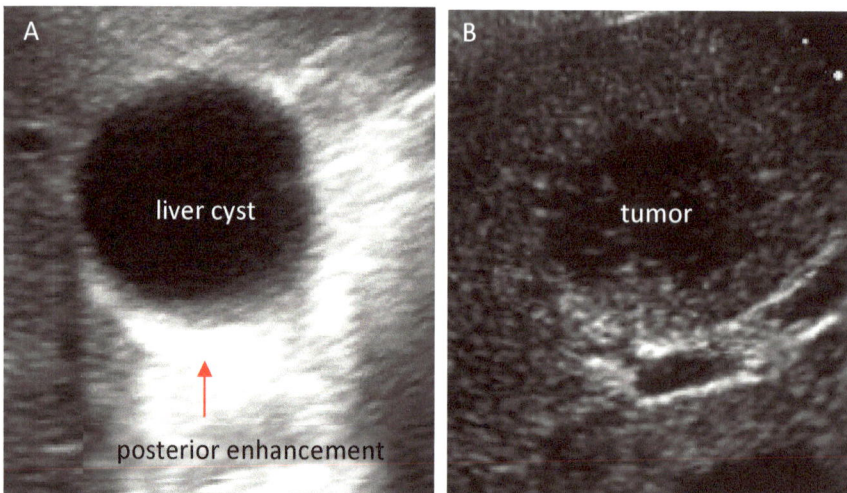

Figure 3.3 Using enhancement artifact to identify structures.
A. Ultrasound image of liver cyst demonstrating posterior enhancement artifact.
B. Ultrasound image of a liver tumor without posterior enhancement artifact.

Disadvantage

The enhancement artifact can introduce error. When measuring the thickness of the gallbladder wall, the posterior wall is "enhanced" and appears thicker than it is. Measuring the posterior wall will overestimate the thickness of the gallbladder wall.

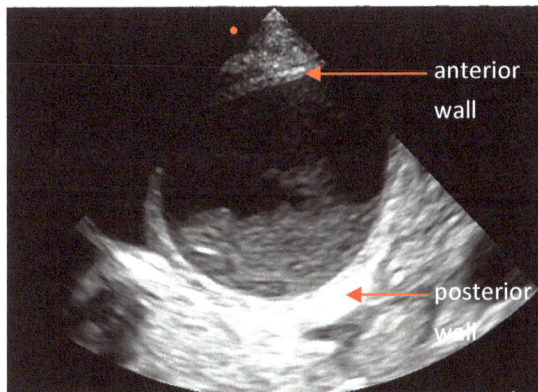

Figure 3.4 Enhancement artifact of posterior gallbladder wall.
Red circle denotes orientation marker.

3.4. Mirror image artifact

When ultrasound encounters a highly reflective curved surface such as the diaphragm, part of the reflected ultrasound travels through the liver and returns directly to the probe. However, part of the ultrasound follows a longer indirect trajectory in returning to the probe. The ultrasound machine can interpret this longer return time as representing a deeper structure. This interpretation can result in a "mirror" image of the liver appearing deep to the diaphragm.

Advantage

A mirror image of the liver will not usually form in the presence of a pleural effusion. The presence of a mirror image of the liver above the diaphragm generally excludes a pleural effusion at that point.

Disadvantage

The mirror image of the liver can be misinterpreted as representing consolidated lung.

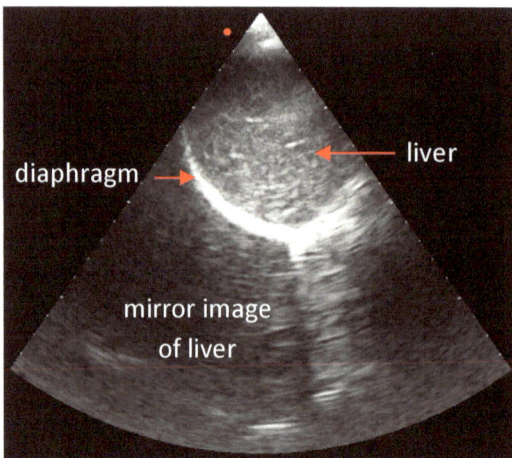

Figure 3.5 Mirror image of the liver below the diaphragm.
Red circle denotes orientation marker.

3.5. Reverberation artifact

When ultrasound encounters two closely apposed reflective surfaces, such as the parietal and visceral pleura, the ultrasound reverberates between the two surfaces. This reverberation creates parallel linear artifacts at equidistant intervals on the ultrasound image.

Advantage

Reverberation artifacts that occur while imaging the lung are called 'A' lines. The presence of 'A' lines on an ultrasound image of the chest can be used in the assessment of a patient with dyspnea (see Chapter 4).

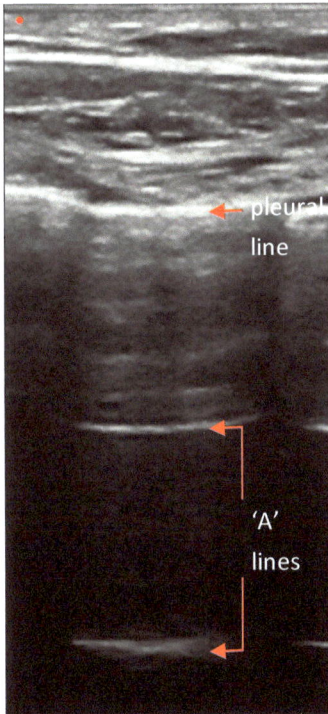

Figure 3.6 'A' lines in a normal lung.

Anterior chest scan with a linear probe. Red circle denotes orientation marker.

3.6. Troubleshooting tips

- When rib shadows obscure the view of the kidney, ask the patient to breathe in and hold their breath. This action will cause the kidney to descend below the ribs and improve the quality of the image.

- The enhancement artifact overestimates the thickness of the posterior gallbladder wall. Therefore measure the thickness of the anterior gallbladder wall instead.

- Mirror image artifacts generally disappear when the orientation of the probe is changed.

- Reverberation artifacts ('A' lines) appear more curved when using a curvilinear or phased array probe.

4. Dyspnea

Case scenario:

A 70 year-old woman presents herself to your clinic complaining of dyspnea. She is too short of breath to provide a useful history. Her respiratory rate is 40 breaths/min, her oxygen saturation is 80%, and she is tachycardic with normal blood pressure. On auscultation, there is poor air entry bilaterally.

Impression: Dyspnea NYD. Consider common causes.

Common causes of **dyspnea** can be recognized by ultrasound examination of the chest. This chapter reviews the technique for diagnosis of pneumothorax, interpretation of lung artifacts, and identification of pleural effusions.

4.1. Probe choice

Both low and high frequency probes can be used for this application.

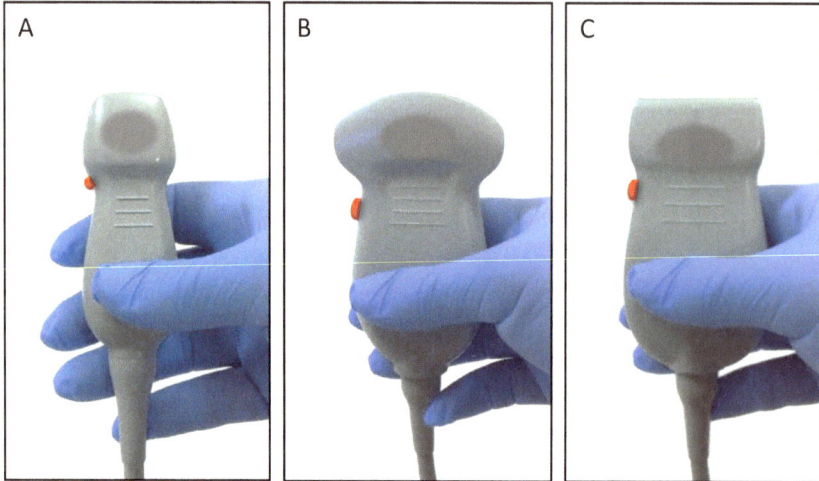

Figure 4.1 Low and high frequency probes that can be used for assessing a patient with dyspnea.

A. A low frequency phased array probe.
B. A low frequency curvilinear probe.
C. A high frequency linear probe. Red circle denotes orientation marker.

4.2. Patient position and scanning technique

The patient should lie supine or be semi-seated in bed. Scan the anterior chest in the second to third rib interspace in the mid-clavicular line and the fourth to fifth rib interspace in the anterior axillary line.

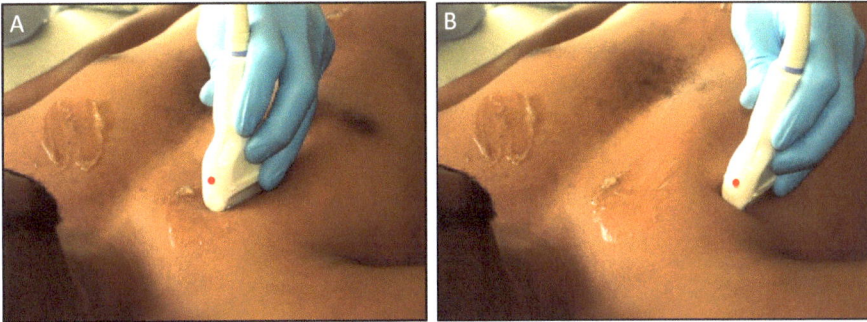

Figure 4.2 Scanning technique for imaging the anterior chest.

*The anterior chest is imaged bilaterally with a linear probe in the mid-clavicular line **(A)** and anterior axillary line **(B)**. The orientation marker points cephalad. Red circle denotes orientation marker.*

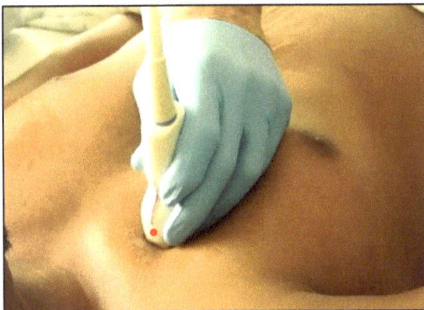

Video 4.1 Scanning technique with lateral rocking motion.

The lateral rocking motion of the probe improves the sensitivity for locating pathology (Lichtenstein, 2010). Red circle denotes orientation marker. View video online at bedsideultrasoundlevel1.com

4.3. Lung sliding

During respiration, the parietal and visceral pleura slide over one another. This horizontal pleural movement during respiration is observed on an ultrasound image and is called **lung sliding** (Lichtenstein et al., 1995).

Characteristics of lung sliding

- The area deep to the pleural line sways side-to-side with the patient's breathing

- The hyperechoic (white) pleural line moves or 'shimmers'

Clinical relevance of lung sliding – Pneumothorax

A pneumothorax is a collection of air between the parietal and visceral pleura. Air in the pleural space prevents the contact between the pleurae and therefore prevents lung sliding. In all cases of pneumothorax, lung sliding will be absent in the scanned area over the anterior chest of a supine patient. Therefore normal lung sliding confidently rules out pneumothorax (Kirkpatrick et al., 2004; Lichtenstein et al., 2005; Noble et al., 2007; Piette et al., 2013).

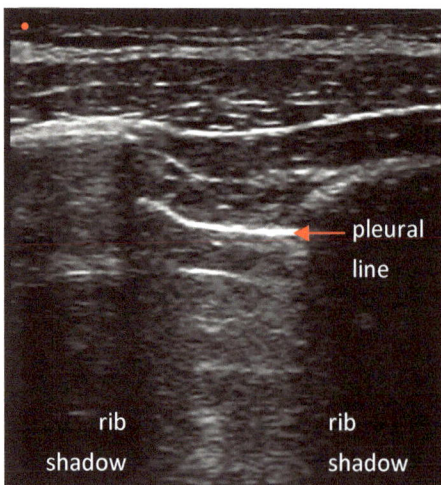

Video 4.2 Presence of lung sliding on the anterior chest using a linear probe.

The hyperechoic (white) pleural line 'shimmers', thus illustrating lung sliding. Accordingly, this patient does not have a pneumothorax. Red circle denotes orientation marker. View video online at bedsideultrasoundlevel1.com

Importantly, the absence of lung sliding **suggests but is not specific** for a pneumothorax because there are other conditions in which lung sliding is absent or hard to detect. These conditions include pleural adhesions, atelectasis, apnea, unilateral bronchial intubation, and extremely shallow rapid breathing (asthma) (Lichtenstein, 2010).

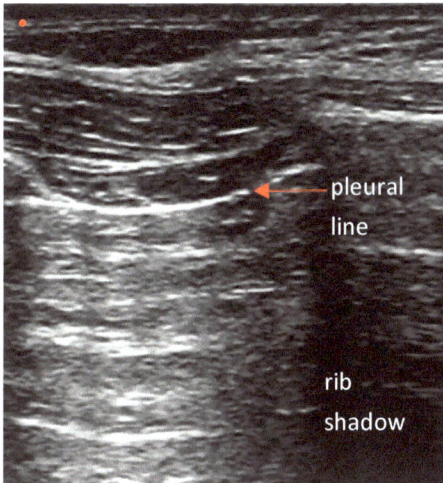

Video 4.3 Absence of lung sliding on the anterior chest using a linear probe.

Note that the pleural line does not 'shimmer' or slide laterally. Therefore, this patient may have a pneumothorax. Red circle denotes orientation marker. View video online at bedsideultrasoundlevel1.com

When the absence of lung sliding is observed, a pneumothorax can be confirmed by detecting a **lung point**. The lung point is an ultrasound landmark specific for a pneumothorax (Lichtenstein et al., 2000).

To look for a lung point, start scanning the anterior chest of a supine patient in whom you have detected the absence of lung sliding. Gradually scan over the chest posterolaterally. A lung point is defined by the alternating presence and absence of lung sliding between two ribs as the patient breathes. The lung point corresponds to that area over the chest wall where the partially deflated lung moves into the ultrasound field of view during inspiration and then out again during expiration.

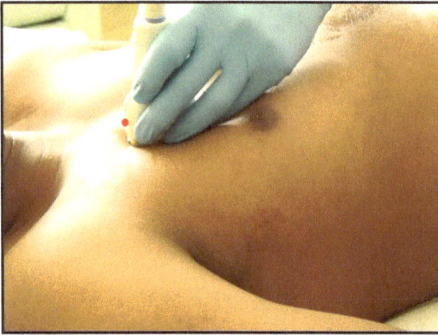

Video 4.4 Scanning technique for imaging a lung point using a linear probe.

Red circle denotes orientation marker. View video online at bedsideultrasoundlevel1.com

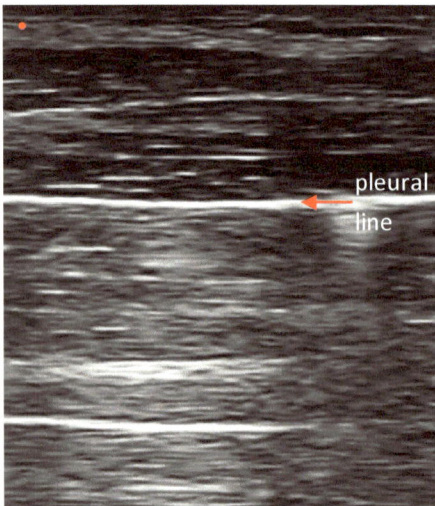

Video 4.5 Lung point on posterolateral chest using linear probe.

Note the lung sliding coming and going from the right of the screen. Red circle denotes orientation marker. View video online at bedsideultrasoundlevel1.com

4.4. 'A' lines

An **'A' line** artifact is a hyperechoic (white) horizontal line arising at regular intervals from the pleural line. An 'A' line artifact is produced when scanning the anterior chest of a patient with normal lungs or in a patient with diseased lungs without interstitial disease (e.g. obstructive airways disease) (Lichtenstein, 2010).

Characteristics of 'A' lines

- Horizontal hyperechoic (white) lines

- Evenly spaced throughout the ultrasound field

- Immobile

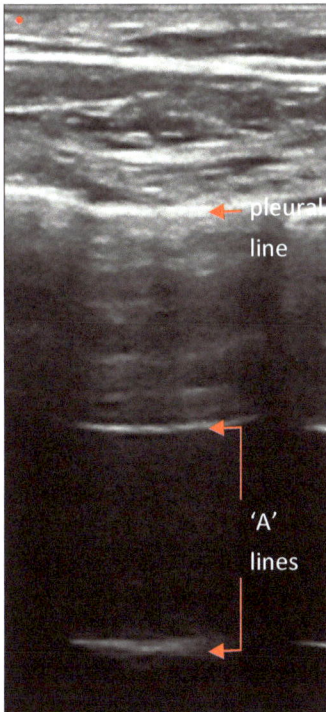

Figure 4.3 'A' lines in a normal lung.

Anterior chest scan with a linear probe. Red circle denotes orientation marker.

4.5. 'B' lines

A **'B' line** artifact is a hyperechoic (white) vertical line arising from the pleural line. A 'B' line is a non-specific artifact produced with any disease of the pulmonary interstitium including pneumonia, pulmonary edema, interstitial fibrosis, and acute respiratory distress syndrome. Three or more 'B' lines between two rib shadows are considered abnormal (Lichtenstein et al., 1998).

Characteristics of 'B' lines

- Vertical, comet-shaped hyperechoic (white) lines

- Originate at the pleura and extend to the far-field of the ultrasound screen

- Move with the pleura

- Eliminate 'A' lines

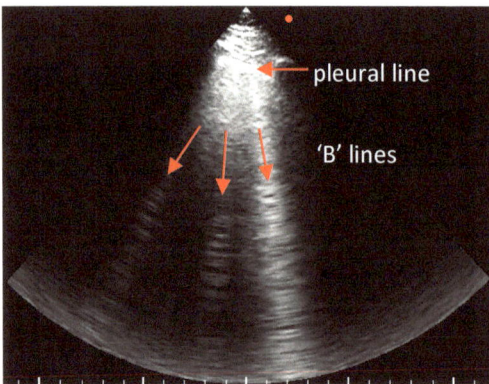

Video 4.6. 'B' lines in a diseased lung.

Anterior chest scan (with a phased array probe in the cardiac setting) displaying vertical 'B' lines that originate at the pleura and extend to the far-field. Red circle denotes orientation marker. View video online at bedsideultrasoundlevel1.com

4.6. Lung profiles

Clinical relevance of 'A' lines - 'A' profile

If you see lung sliding with 'A' lines on bilateral anterior chest exams, the patient is defined as having an **'A' profile.** Patients presenting with an 'A' profile and dyspnea generally have chronic obstructive pulmonary disease (COPD) or asthma exacerbation. Patients with an 'A' profile, dyspnea, and a deep venous thrombosis (DVT) are likely to have a pulmonary embolism (Lichtenstein et al., 2008).

Clinical relevance of 'B' lines - 'B' profile

If you see lung sliding with 'B' lines on bilateral anterior chest scans, the patient is defined as having a **'B' profile**. Dyspneic patients presenting to the emergency room with a 'B' profile generally have cardiogenic pulmonary edema (Lichtenstein and Meziere, 2008).

However, the interpretation of lung profiles must always be done in context of the clinical impression. For example, a patient presenting with a 'B' profile in association with fever, rigors, cough, and productive sputum, likely has bilateral pneumonia and not cardiogenic pulmonary edema.

Clinical relevance of 'A' + 'B' lines - 'AB' profile

If one side of the anterior chest has 'A' lines while the other side has 'B' lines the patient is said to have an **'AB' profile.** Patients presenting with an 'AB' profile and dyspnea are likely to have pneumonia as the cause of their dyspnea (Lichtenstein and Meziere, 2008).

Table 4.1 Lung profiles and common associated pathologies in outpatients presenting with dyspnea.

Lung profile	Pathology
'A' lines 'A' lines 'A' profile	COPD Asthma Pulmonary embolism (if DVT present)
'B' lines 'B' lines 'B' profile	Cardiogenic pulmonary edema
'A' lines 'B' lines 'AB' profile	Pneumonia

4.7. Posterolateral chest

The posterolateral chest is examined for pleural effusions and lung consolidation.

Characteristics of the posterolateral chest exam

- Diaphragm appears as a hyperechoic (white) line, concave caudally
- Normal lung appears as a **'curtain' sign** sweeping into the field as the diaphragm descends
- Pleural effusion appears as an anechoic (black) area above the diaphragm
- Lung consolidation appears as a hypoechoic (grey) structure above the diaphragm

Clinical relevance - Posterolateral chest exam

- Patients with dyspnea, a normal anterior chest exam (bilateral 'A' lines), no DVT, and an unilateral pleural effusion or consolidation, likely have pneumonia (Lichtenstein and Meziere, 2008)
- Patients with left ventricular dysfunction, a 'B' profile, and bilateral pleural effusions likely have congestive heart failure (Lichtenstein and Meziere, 2008)
- Pleural effusions with hyperechoic (white) floating particles or septae are likely to be exudative (Yang et al., 1992)
- Ultrasound can be used to safely guide a thoracentesis (Barnes et al., 2005; Jones et al., 2003)

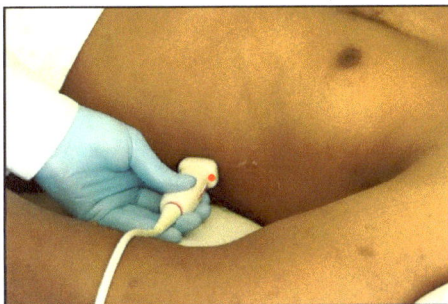

Video 4.7 Scanning technique for imaging a pleural effusion or lung consolidation over the left posterolateral chest using a phased array probe.

Red circle denotes orientation marker. View video online at bedsideultrasoundlevel1.com

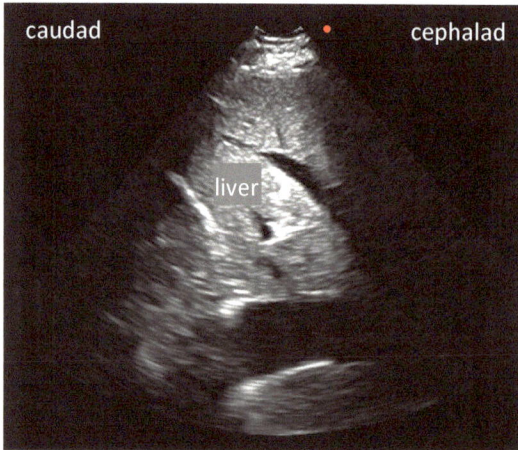

caudad cephalad

liver

Video 4.8 Normal lung revealed by a posterolateral chest scan with a phased array probe in the cardiac setting.

As the diaphragm descends caudally, the lung enters the right-side field of view. This is termed the 'curtain' sign. Red circle denotes orientation marker. View video online at bedsideultrasoundlevel1.com

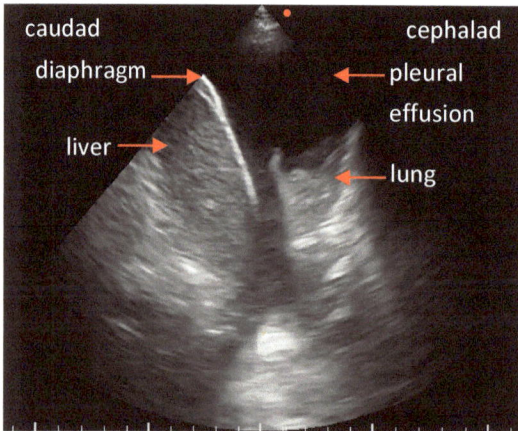

caudad cephalad
diaphragm pleural effusion
liver lung

Video 4.9 Large pleural effusion revealed by a posterolateral chest scan with a phased array probe in the cardiac setting.

The pleural effusion is cephalad to the diaphragm and appears anechoic (black). Red circle denotes orientation marker. View video online at bedsideultrasoundlevel1.com

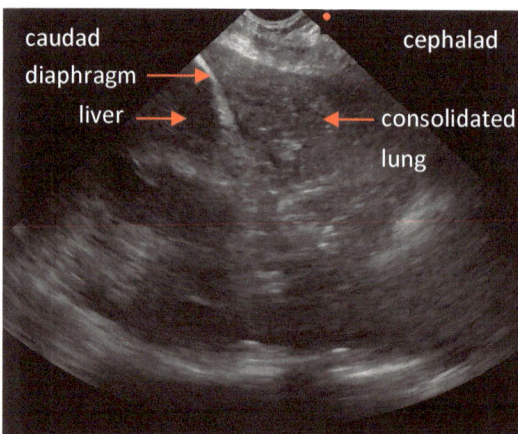

caudad cephalad
diaphragm
liver consolidated lung

Figure 4.4 Lung consolidation revealed by a posterolateral chest scan with a phased array probe in the cardiac setting.

The consolidated lung is a hypoechoic (grey) structure. Red circle denotes orientation marker.

4.8. Troubleshooting tips

- To detect a pneumothorax in a supine patient, be sure to examine the anterior chest. This is because the pneumothorax will accumulate anteriorly.

- Beware that a lung point will not be found in a tension pneumothorax because the lung is completely collapsed in this condition and therefore does not contact the chest wall.

- In cachectic patients with a protruding rib cage, it is difficult to establish adequate contact between a linear probe and the chest wall. This difficulty can be overcome by turning the probe in the transverse plane so that it fits between the ribs, or by using a microconvex probe.

- If lung sliding is difficult to identify with a low frequency probe, use a linear high frequency probe instead.

Case closed:

The 70 year-old woman who presented herself to your clinic complaining of dyspnea has clinical evidence of congestive heart failure. She is found to have a 'B' profile on lung ultrasound. Diuretic is administered and the patient is hospitalized.

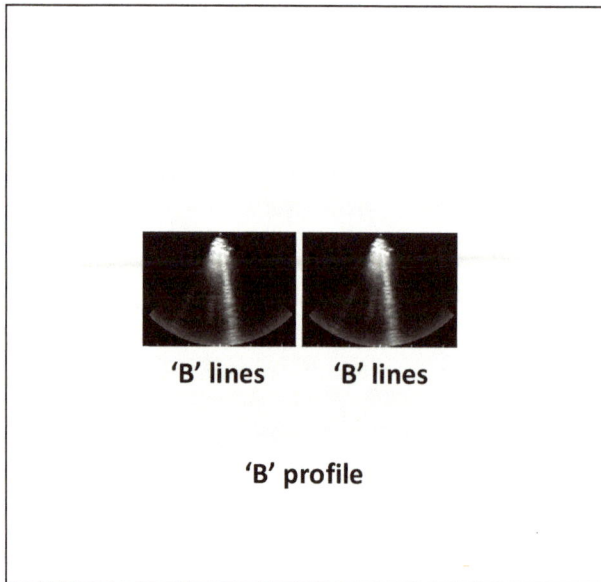

'B' lines   'B' lines

'B' profile

Patient with a 'B' profile has 'B' lines on bilateral anterior chest scans.

5. Undifferentiated hypotension

Case scenario:

An 80 year-old man is found unconscious in his home, and no medical history is available. At the hospital, he is hypotensive with a blood pressure of 70/40 mmHg, and a heart rate of 120 beats/min. He is normothermic, breathing shallowly at 30 breaths/min, and his oxygen saturation is unobtainable. His neck veins are not visible. He has poor air entry bilaterally and some tenderness on abdominal exam. No bowel sounds are present. His legs are mottled.

Impression: Undifferentiated hypotension. Consider common causes.

Bedside ultrasound can help to identify certain causes of **undifferentiated hypotension**. This chapter introduces the ultrasonographic signs associated with left ventricular dysfunction, massive pulmonary embolism, tamponade, and hypovolemia.

5.1. Probe choice

A low frequency phased array probe is commonly used for this application, however a low frequency curvilinear probe is also an appropriate choice.

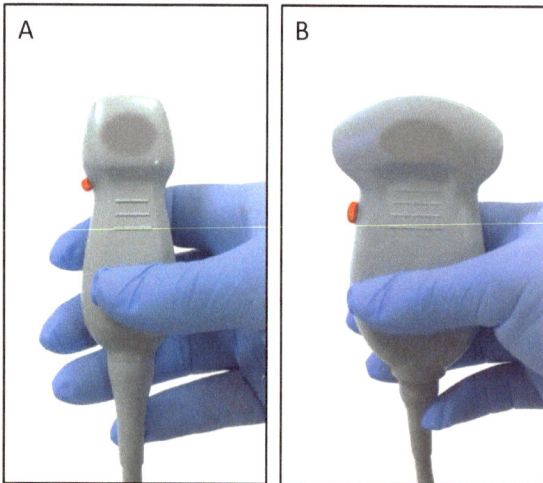

Figure 5.1 Low frequency probes that can be used for assessing a patient with undifferentiated hypotension.

A. A phased array probe.
B. A curvilinear probe. Red circle denotes orientation marker.

5.2. Patient position and scanning technique

This application is best performed with the patient in the supine position.

5.3. Left ventricular function

Estimating left ventricular (LV) function can help distinguish between different causes of hypotension. To estimate LV function, obtain a subxiphoid view of the heart by placing the phased array probe in the subxiphoid area with the orientation marker pointing to the patient's left.

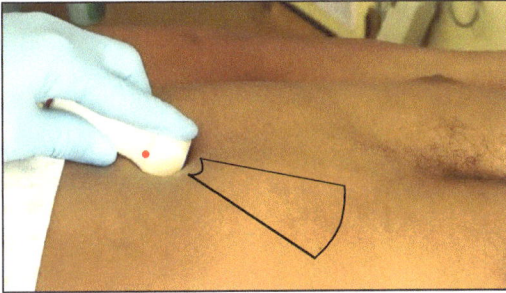

Video 5.1 Scanning technique to obtain a subxiphoid view of the heart.

Red circle denotes orientation marker. View video online at bedsideultrasoundlevel1.com

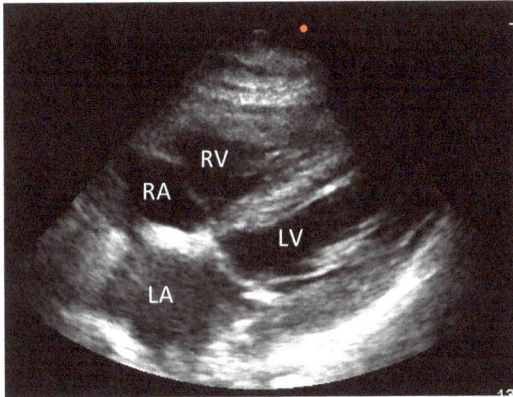

Figure 5.2 Subxiphoid view of the heart.

Subxiphoid view of the heart demonstrating the four chambers.
LV: left ventricle, LA: left atrium, RA: right atrium, RV: right ventricle. Red circle denotes orientation marker.

On the ultrasound image of a normal heart during systole, the LV walls thicken, and the LV diameter decreases by 30%. The LV diameter is measured from inner wall to inner wall. The measurement is made one third of the way from the mitral valve annulus to the apex. The decrease in LV diameter during systole is termed '**fractional shortening**' (Anderson, 2000).

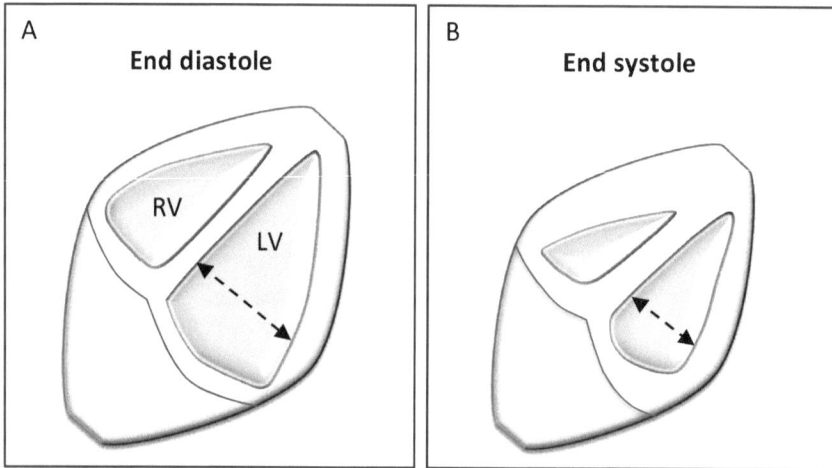

Figure 5.3 Measuring left ventricular (LV) diameter.
LV diameter is measured from inner wall to inner wall.
A. LV diameter at the end of diastole.
B. LV diameter decreases by 30% during normal systole.
RV: Right ventricle.

LV function can also be assessed using a subjective visual estimate of the change in LV size between systole and diastole (Amico et al., 1989; Mueller et al., 1991; Randazzo et al., 2003; Stamm et al., 1982).

The following four videos illustrate different categories of LV function.

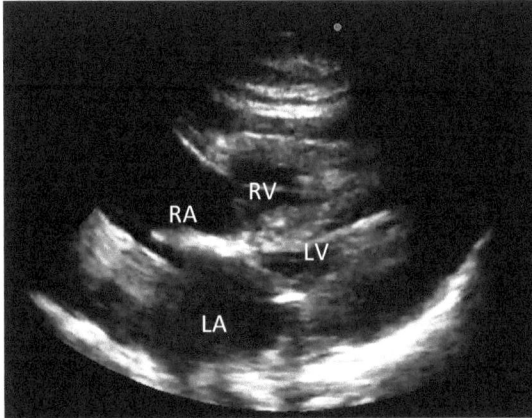

Video 5.2 Hyperdynamic LV function in the subxiphoid view.

LV: left ventricle, LA: left atrium, RA: right atrium, RV: right ventricle. Red circle denotes orientation marker. View video online at bedsideultrasoundlevel1.com

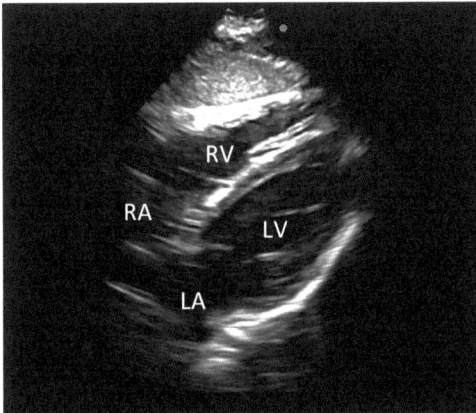

Video 5.3 Normal LV function in the subxiphoid view.

LV: left ventricle, LA: left atrium, RA: right atrium, RV: right ventricle. Red circle denotes orientation marker. View video online at bedsideultrasoundlevel1.com

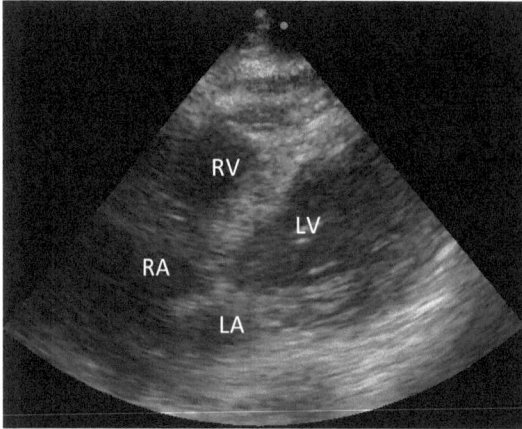

Video 5.4 Moderate LV dysfunction in the subxiphoid view.

LV: left ventricle, LA: left atrium, RA: right atrium, RV: right ventricle. Red circle denotes orientation marker. View video online at bedsideultrasoundlevel1.com

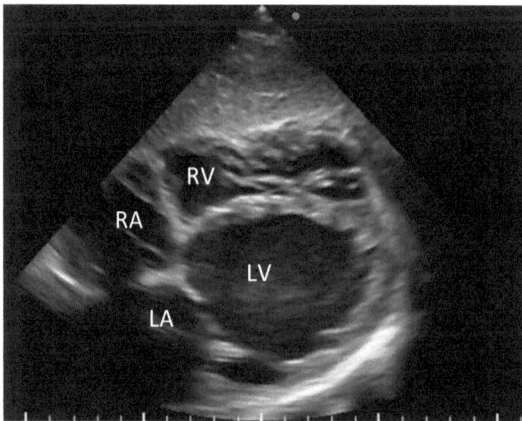

Video 5.5 Severe LV dysfunction in the subxiphoid view.

LV: left ventricle, LA: left atrium, RA: right atrium, RV: right ventricle. Red circle denotes orientation marker. View video online at bedsideultrasoundlevel1.com

LV function can be classified into three categories: hyperdynamic, normal, and LV dysfunction (mild, moderate, and severe).

Table 5.1 Categories and characteristics of left ventricular (LV) function.

Categories of LV function	Ultrasound image characteristics
Hyperdynamic LV function	Tachycardia Thickening of ventricular walls during systole Apposition or 'kissing' of ventricular walls during systole
Normal LV function	Thickening of ventricular walls during systole Fractional shortening of LV diameter by 30% during systole
Mild to moderate to severe LV dysfunction	Progressive decreases in: • wall thickening during systole • wall motion during systole • fractional shortening of LV diameter during systole

Clinical relevance - LV function

In a hypotensive patient:

- Hyperdynamic LV function is consistent with hypovolemia as a cause of the hypotension (e.g. bleeding) among other diagnoses (see Table 5.2)

- Moderate and severe LV dysfunction are consistent with a cardiogenic cause for the hypotension (e.g. myocardial infarction)

5.4. Right to left ventricular diameter ratio

Normally the right ventricular (RV) chamber diameter should not exceed 60% of the LV chamber diameter at the end of diastole. Thus the RV to LV diameter ratio equals 0.6 (RV:LV ratio ≤ 0.6) (Jardin et al., 1997). RV chamber diameter is measured from inner wall to inner wall (Anderson, 2000).

The RV diameter increases acutely with massive pulmonary emboli due to an abrupt rise in the right ventricular afterload (Reardon et al., 2008).

Clinical relevance - Pulmonary embolism

In a hypotensive patient with a suspected pulmonary embolism:

- An acute increase in the RV:LV ratio supports the suspicion of a pulmonary embolism as a cause of hypotension

- A normal RV:LV ratio does not rule out pulmonary embolism, but makes massive pulmonary embolism as the sole cause of hypotension unlikely

Caution is warranted before attributing an increased RV:LV ratio to pulmonary embolism. An increase in the RV:LV ratio can be seen in other acute (pneumonia, acute respiratory distress syndrome) and chronic (chronic obstructive pulmonary disease) conditions (Jackson et al., 2000).

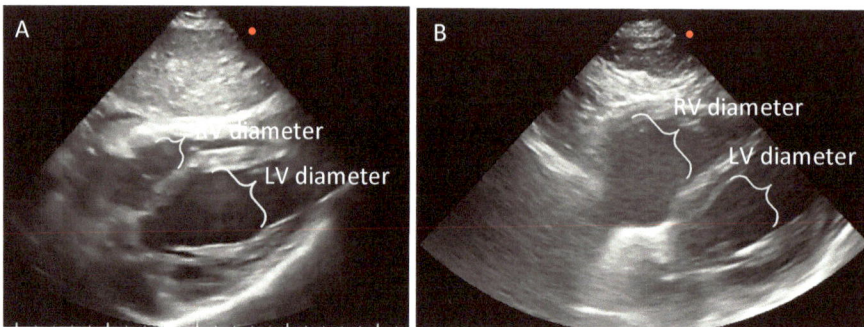

Figure 5.4 Right to left ventricular diameter ratio in a subxiphoid view of the heart.
A. Normal right ventricular (RV) to left ventricular (LV) diameter ratio (≤ 0.6).
B. Increased RV:LV (>0.6). Red circle denotes orientation marker.

5.5. Pericardial effusion

A pericardial effusion is a collection of fluid between the parietal and visceral pericardium. The pericardial effusion will appear as an anechoic (black) area around the heart. When a pericardial effusion reduces heart chamber compliance and leads to a decrease in venous return, cardiac output, and blood pressure, this is termed **cardiac tamponade** (Reardon and Joing, 2008).

Clinical relevance – Cardiac tamponade

In a hypotensive patient:

- The presence of a pericardial effusion raises the possibility that cardiac tamponade is present

- The absence of pericardial effusion excludes cardiac tamponade

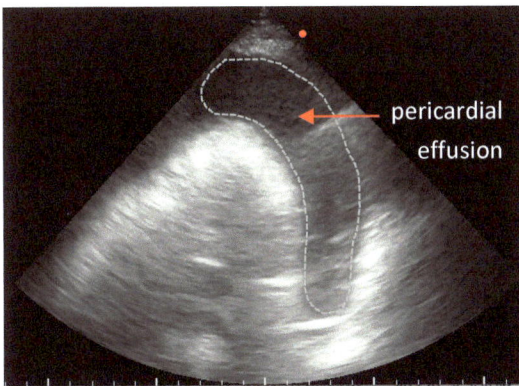

Video 5.6 A large pericardial effusion in the subxiphoid view.

The heart chambers are collapsed due to the pericardial effusion. This patient has tamponade. Red circle denotes orientation marker. View video online at bedsideultrasoundlevel1.com

5.6. Volume status and the IVC

Vascular volume depletion (**hypovolemia**) is one of the causes of hypotension. Volume status can be assessed with ultrasound imaging of the diameter of the inferior vena cava (IVC) and its respiratory variability.

Respiratory variability describes the decrease in IVC diameter as a spontaneously breathing patient inspires.

The diameter and respiratory variability of the IVC are measured 3-4 cm proximal to the right atrial-IVC junction (Lyon et al., 2005; Natori et al., 1979; Simonson et al., 1988).

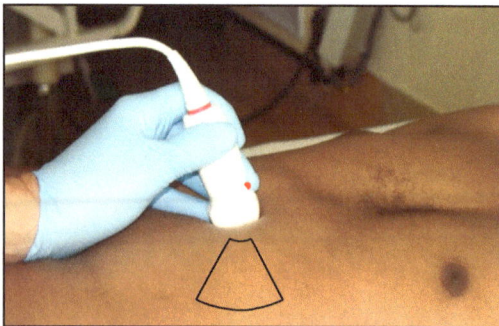

Figure 5.5 Scanning technique for imaging the inferior vena cava (IVC).

A phased array probe is placed in the subxiphoid area with the orientation marker pointing cephalad to image the IVC in the sagittal plane. Red circle denotes orientation marker.

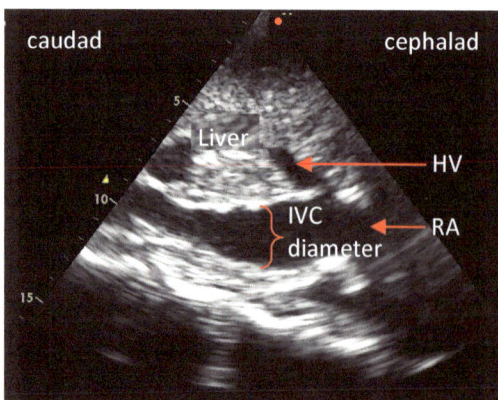

Figure 5.6 Sagittal view of the inferior vena cava (IVC).

The phased array probe is used here in the 'cardiac setting' hence the orientation marker is on the upper right hand side. HV: hepatic vein, RA: right atrium. Red circle denotes orientation marker.

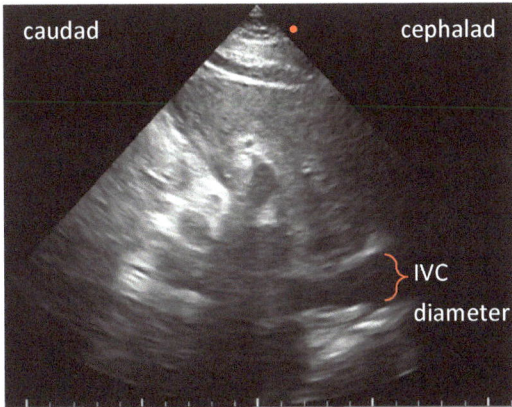

Video 5.7 Significant respiratory variability of the inferior vena cava (IVC).

Sagittal view of the IVC showing how the diameter of the IVC varies during respiration. In this example, there is complete collapse of the IVC.
Red circle denotes orientation marker. View video online at bedsideultrasoundlevel1.com

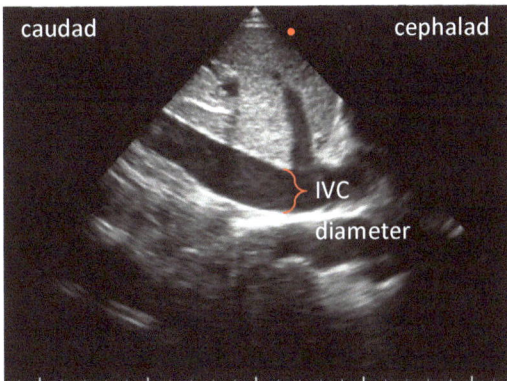

Video 5.8 Minimal respiratory variability of the inferior vena cava (IVC).

Sagittal view of the IVC showing a lack of IVC diameter respiratory variability.
Red circle denotes orientation marker. View video online at bedsideultrasoundlevel1.com

Studies have shown some correlation of a patient's volume status with both IVC diameter and its respiratory variability (Kircher et al., 1990; Ommen et al., 2000; Simonson and Schiller, 1988; Wong, 2002).

Clinical relevance

In a hypotensive patient:

- When hypovolemia is the cause of the hypotension, the IVC diameter is generally <15 mm and varies more than 50% with respiration

- The initial treatment usually involves an infusion of a volume expander (e.g. NS or Ringer's lactate). The effect of volume infusion can be evaluated with serial monitoring of the IVC diameter and respiratory variability. For example, adequate volume infusion given to a hypovolemic patient should increase the diameter and decrease the variability of the IVC (Reardon and Joing, 2008)

- When either myocardial infarction, pulmonary embolism, or tamponade is the cause of the hypotension, the IVC diameter is generally >20 mm and varies less than 50% with respiration

Table 5.2 Summary table of the common causes of hypotension and their bedside ultrasound findings.

Causes of hypotension	IVC diameter / variability	LV function
Myocardial infarction	Large and not variable	Moderate or severe LV dysfunction
Pulmonary embolism	Large and not variable	Hyperdynamic LV function with increased RV:LV ratio
Tamponade	Large and not variable	Small cardiac chambers with hyperdynamic LV function and pericardial effusion
Hypovolemia	Small and variable	Hyperdynamic LV function
Sepsis	Commonly small and variable but may be increased with associated LV dysfunction	Commonly hyperdynamic LV function but may see moderate or severe LV dysfunction in later stages

5.7. Additional ultrasound assessments for hypotension

Additional focused bedside ultrasound examinations can help determine the cause of hypotension following the assessment of the LV function, RV:LV ratio, pericardium, and IVC.

For example:

- If tension pneumothorax is suspected, look for the absence of lung sliding (Chapter 4)

- If intraabdominal bleeding is suspected in trauma, look for free intraabdominal fluid (Chapter 6)

- If abdominal pain is present, look for an AAA (Chapter 7)

- If ectopic pregnancy is suspected, look for the absence of intrauterine pregnancy (Chapter 11)

5.8. Troubleshooting tips

- If the heart is difficult to visualize in the subxiphoid view, ask the patient to breathe in and hold their breath. This action can bring the heart closer to the probe and provide a better image.

- When imaging the IVC, apply light pressure on the probe. Excessive pressure will collapse the IVC.

- In a patient receiving positive pressure ventilation, the IVC diameter increases rather than decreases during inspiration.

- A pericardial fat pad can be confused with a pericardial effusion. Pericardial fat pads are hypoechoic (grey) and not anechoic (black).

Case closed:

The 80 year-old hypotensive man has a hyperdynamic LV, normal RV:LV ratio, no pericardial effusion, and a small variable IVC, suggesting hypovolemia. As volume expanders are administered, further ultrasound examination reveals a large ruptured abdominal aortic aneurysm. A vascular surgeon is urgently consulted.

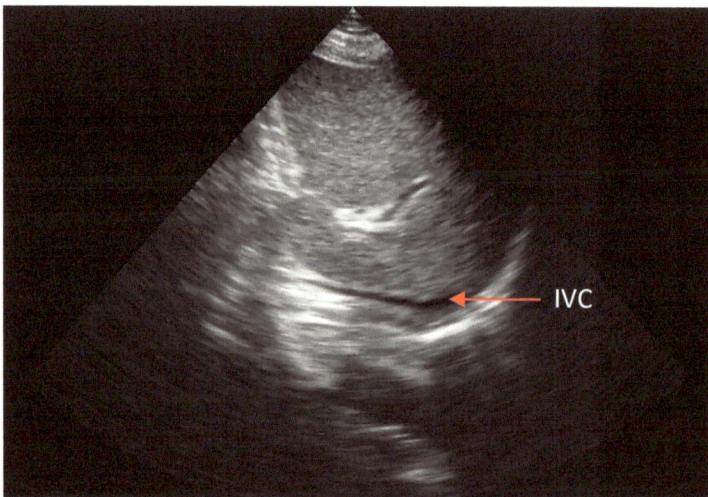

Sagittal view of a small diameter IVC.

6. Trauma

Case scenario:

A 25 year-old woman is struck by a car and is brought to the emergency room by ambulance. She is conscious, and complains of abdominal and chest pain. Her blood pressure is 80/60 mmHg, and her heart rate is 120 beats/min. Her abdomen is tender without peritoneal signs.

Impression: Hypotension in the setting of trauma. Rule out intraabdominal bleeding.

This chapter will introduce the use of bedside ultrasound in diagnosing intraabdominal bleeding, hemopericardium, hemothorax, and pneumothorax in the setting of trauma.

6.1. Probe choice

A low frequency curvilinear probe is commonly used for this application, however a phased array probe in the abdominal setting is also an appropriate choice.

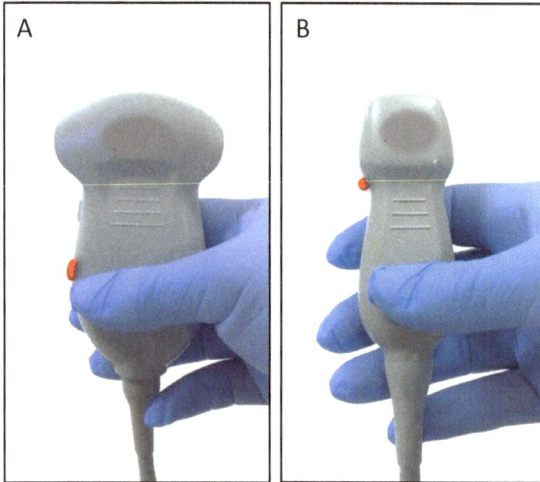

Figure 6.1 Low frequency probes that can be used for assessing a trauma patient.
A. *A phased array probe.*
B. *A curvilinear probe. Red circle denotes orientation marker.*

6.2. Patient position and scanning technique

Patients are evaluated in the supine position.

6.3. The eFAST algorithm

Bedside ultrasound is useful in answering four questions in the setting of trauma (Noble, Nelson et al., 2007):

Question #1: Does the patient have free intraabdominal or pelvic fluid?
>In the trauma patient, free intraabdominal or pelvic fluid is assumed to be blood until proven otherwise.

Question #2: Does the patient have a hemopericardium?
>In the setting of penetrating thoracic trauma, pericardial fluid is assumed to be blood until proven otherwise.

Question #3: Does the patient have a hemothorax?
>In the trauma patient, a pleural effusion is assumed to be a hemothorax until proven otherwise.

Question #4: Does the patient have a pneumothorax?

These questions can be answered using the **eFAST** algorithm.

The eFAST acronym represents:	e	=	extended
	F	=	Focused
	A	=	Assessment
	S	=	Sonography
	T	=	Trauma

The use of this approach in trauma patients is well supported by the medical literature (Ma et al., 2008; Noble, Nelson et al., 2007; Tayal et al., 2006). This chapter provides a summary of the eFAST algorithm at the introductory level.

Question #1: Does the patient have free intraabdominal or pelvic fluid?

The presence of free intraabdominal or pelvic fluid can be detected by scanning the following three areas:

Area #1: Morison's pouch

Area #2: The spleno-renal space

Area #3: The pelvis

Area #1: Morison's pouch is the potential space between the liver and the upper pole of the right kidney. This space is one of the first places in the abdomen in which free fluid accumulates. To locate free fluid in Morison's pouch, the probe is held on the mid-axillary line at the right 7th-9th intercostal space, with the orientation marker pointing cephalad (Ma and Mateer, 2008; Noble, Nelson et al., 2007; Tayal and Kendall, 2006).

The probe is moved cephalad to caudad in the coronal plane, enabling the examiner to visualize Morison's pouch.

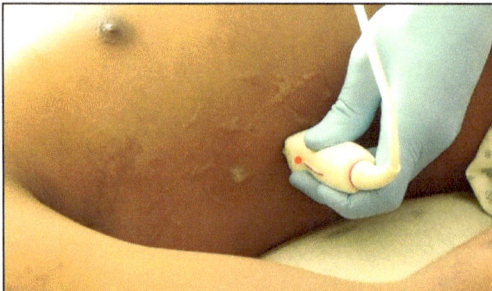

Video 6.1 Scanning technique for imaging free fluid in Morison's pouch using a phased array probe.

Red circle denotes orientation marker. View video online at bedsideultrasoundlevel1.com

The presence of free fluid in Morison's pouch will appear anechoic (black) on the ultrasound image.

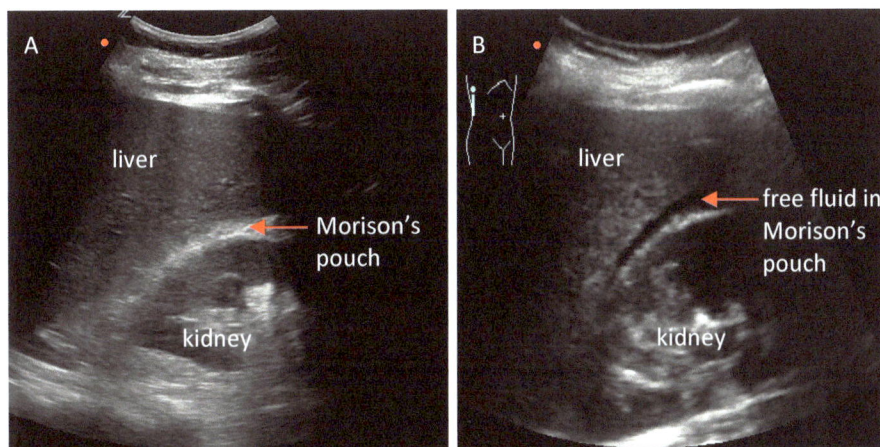

Figure 6.2 Fluid in Morison's pouch revealed by a right posterolateral abdominal scan.

A. The normal appearance of Morison's pouch. There is no anechoic (black) area between the liver and the right kidney.

B. Free fluid in Morison's pouch appears anechoic (black). Red circle denotes orientation marker.

Area #2: The spleno-renal space is the potential space between the spleen and the upper pole of the left kidney. To locate free fluid in the spleno-renal space, the probe is held in the left mid- to posterior-axillary line between the 5th-7th intercostal space with the orientation marker pointing cephalad (Ma and Mateer, 2008; Noble, Nelson et al., 2007; Tayal and Kendall, 2006). The presence of free fluid between the spleen and the left kidney will appear anechoic (black) on the ultrasound image.

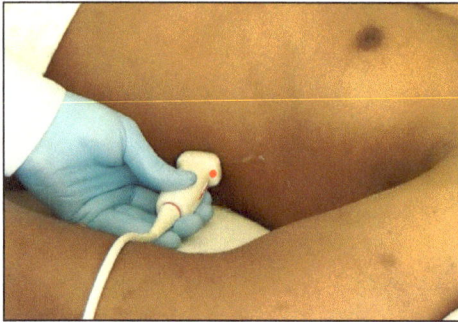

Video 6.2 Scanning technique for imaging free fluid in the spleno-renal space using a phased array probe.

Red circle denotes orientation marker. View video online at bedsideultrasoundlevel1.com

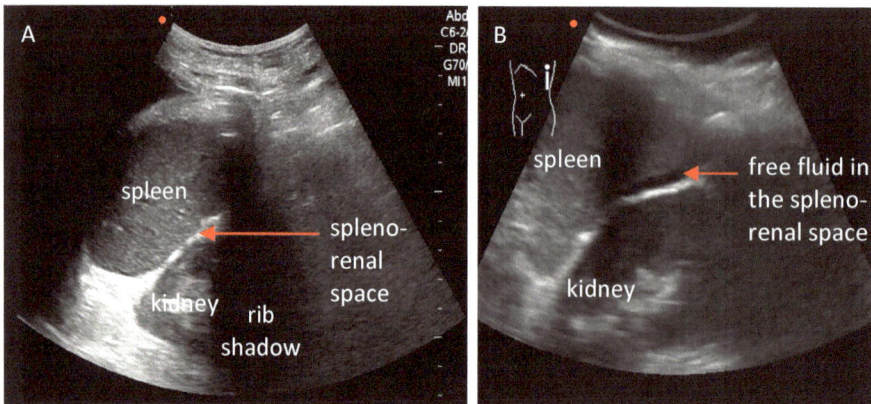

Figure 6.3 Fluid in the spleno-renal space revealed by a left posterolateral abdominal scan.

A. *The normal appearance of the spleno-renal space.*
B. *Free fluid between the spleen and the left kidney appears anechoic (black). Red circle denotes orientation marker.*

Area #3: The pelvis. In females, free pelvic fluid collects in **the pouch of Douglas**. The pouch of Douglas is the potential space between the uterus and the rectum. Women of childbearing age can have a small amount of fluid in this space. In males, free pelvic fluid collects between the bladder and the rectum. To locate free fluid in the pelvis, the probe is placed superior to the symphysis pubis and pointed caudally (Ma and Mateer, 2008; Noble, Nelson et al., 2007; Tayal and Kendall, 2006).

To scan the pelvis in the transverse plane, place the probe just superior to the symphysis pubis with the orientation marker pointing to the patient's right. Sweep the probe caudally. The presence of free fluid will appear anechoic (black) on the ultrasound image.

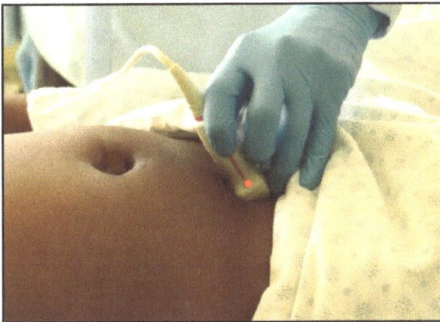

Figure 6.4 Scanning technique for imaging the pelvis in the transverse plane using a phased array probe.

Red circle denotes orientation marker.

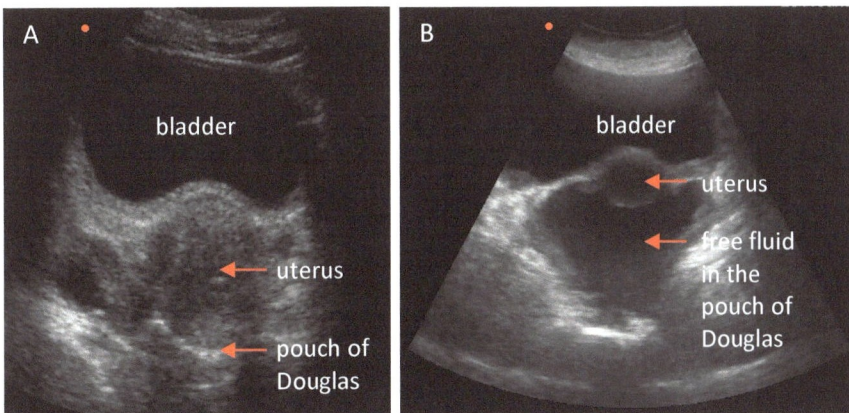

Figure 6.5 The female pelvis in the transverse plane.
A. *The female pelvis without fluid in the pouch of Douglas.*
B. *The female pelvis with free fluid in the pouch of Douglas. Red circle denotes orientation marker.*

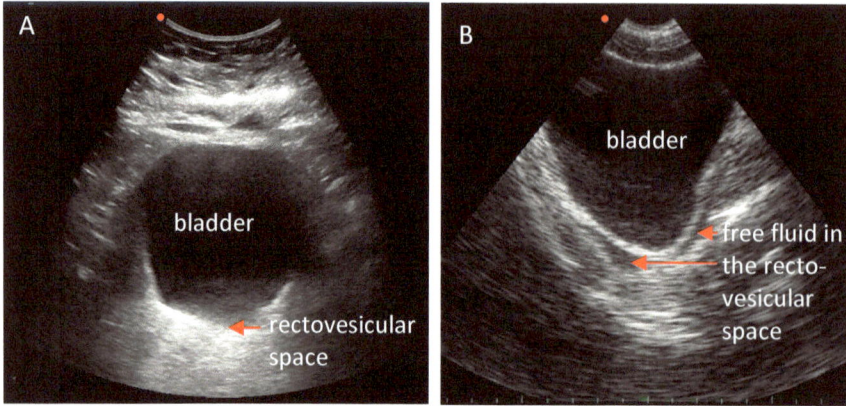

Figure 6.6 The male pelvis in the transverse plane.
A. *The male pelvis without fluid in the rectovesicular space.*
B. *The male pelvis with free fluid in the rectovesicular space. Red circle denotes orientation marker.*

To scan the pelvis in the sagittal plane, place the probe just superior to the symphysis pubis with the orientation marker pointing cephalad. Point the probe caudally.

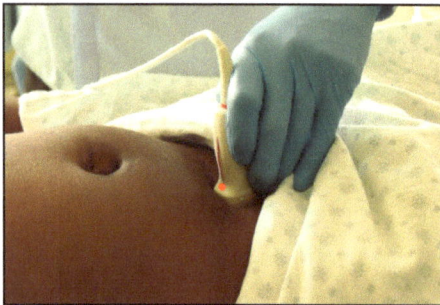

Figure 6.7 Scanning technique for imaging the pelvis in the sagittal plane using a phased array probe.

Red circle denotes orientation marker.

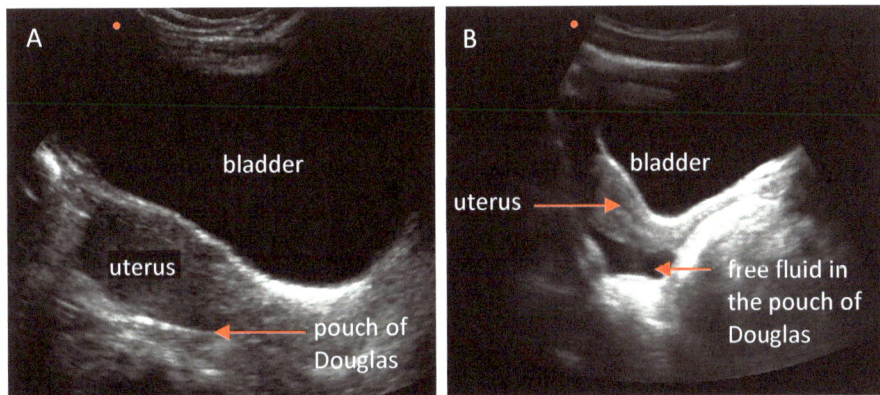

Figure 6.8 The female pelvis in the sagittal plane.
A. The female pelvis in sagittal plane without fluid in the pouch of Douglas.
B. The female pelvis in sagittal plane with free fluid in the pouch of Douglas.
Red circle denotes orientation marker.

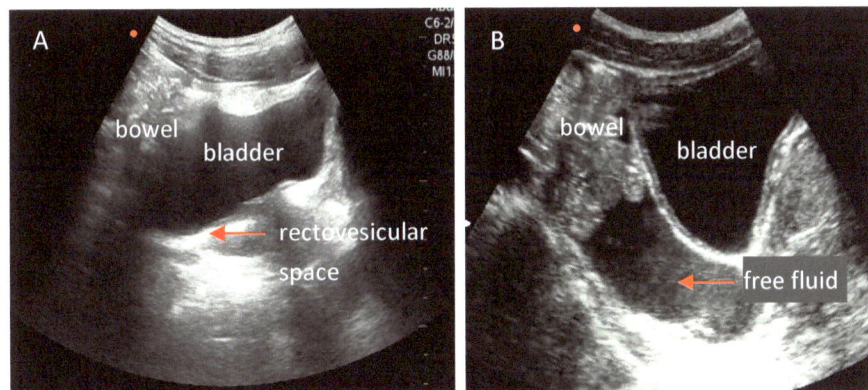

Figure 6.9 The male pelvis in the sagittal plane.
A. The male pelvis in sagittal plane without fluid in the rectovesicular space.
B. The male pelvis in sagittal plane with free fluid in the rectovesicular space.
Red circle denotes orientation marker.

Summary: If a trauma patient has free fluid in…

Area #1: Morison's pouch

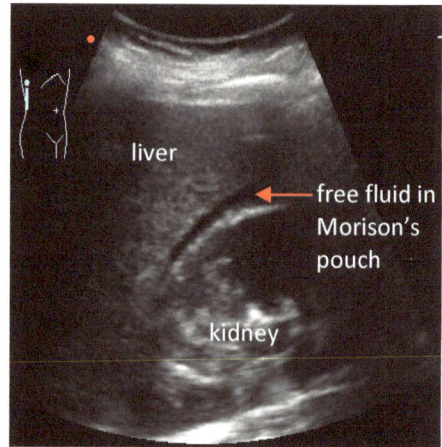

liver

free fluid in Morison's pouch

kidney

Area #2: The spleno-renal space

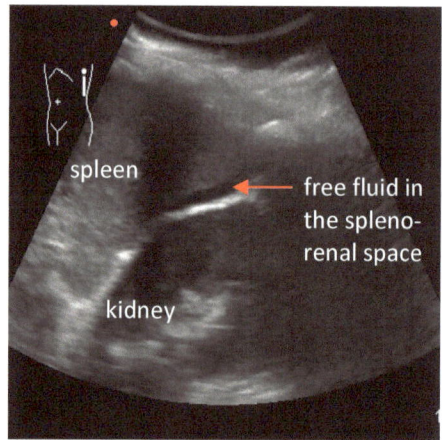

spleen

free fluid in the spleno-renal space

kidney

Area #3: The pelvis

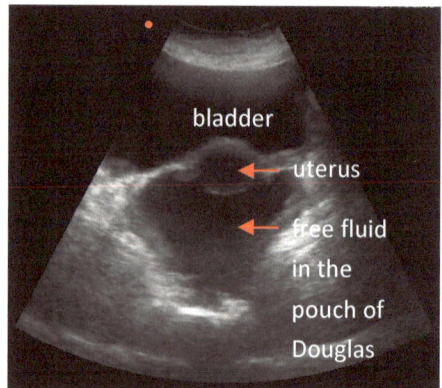

bladder

uterus

free fluid in the pouch of Douglas

…then the clinician suspects intraperitoneal bleeding.

Question #2: Does the patient have a hemopericardium?

In the trauma patient, pericardial fluid is assumed to be blood until proven otherwise.

To look for pericardial fluid, image the heart using the subxiphoid view.

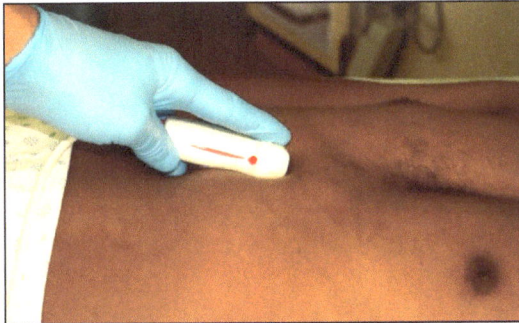

Figure 6.10 Scanning technique for imaging pericardial fluid using the subxiphoid view.

The orientation marker on the phased array probe points to the patient's left.

When using a curvilinear probe in the abdominal setting, the orientation marker points to the patient's right. Red circle denotes orientation marker.

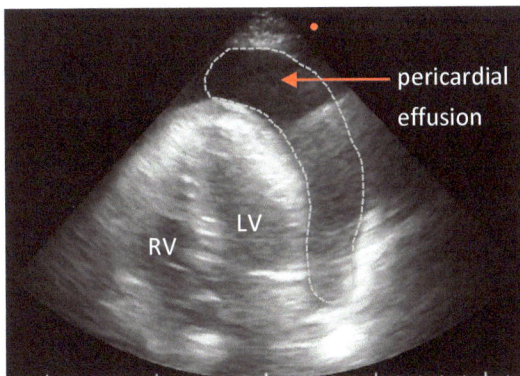

Figure 6.11 A pericardial effusion seen in the subxiphoid view.

The pericardial effusion appears as an anechoic (black) area around the heart. Red circle denotes orientation marker.

Question #3: Does the patient have a hemothorax?

In the trauma patient, a pleural effusion is assumed to be a hemothorax until proven otherwise.

Pleural effusions develop posteriorly in a supine patient. To look for a pleural effusion, scan the posterolateral chest bilaterally. Move the probe in the coronal plane between the posterior and mid-axillary line. Point the orientation marker cephalad.

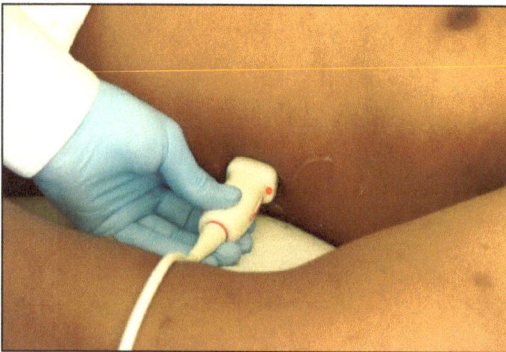

Figure 6.12 Scanning technique for imaging a hemothorax in the left posterolateral chest with a phased array probe.

Red circle denotes orientation marker.

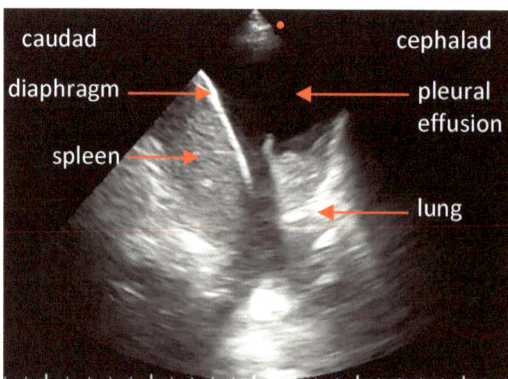

Figure 6.13 A pleural effusion seen in a left posterolateral chest scan.

The pleural effusion appears as an anechoic (black) area above the diaphragm. Red circle denotes orientation marker.

Question #4: Does the patient have a pneumothorax?

A pneumothorax is common in the setting of major trauma. A pneumothorax is the accumulation of air between the parietal and visceral pleurae.

In a supine patient, a pneumothorax accumulates anteriorly and thus an anterior chest scan is essential. In the setting of trauma:

- The presence of lung sliding on an anterior chest exam of a supine patient rules out a pneumothorax (Chapter 4)

- The absence of lung sliding suggests a pneumothorax on the side that was scanned (Chapter 4)

The identification of a pneumothorax on an ultrasound image is explained in detail in Section 4.3 (Kirkpatrick, Sirois et al., 2004; Lichtenstein, Meziere et al., 2005; Noble, Nelson et al., 2007; Ouellet et al., 2011).

6.4. Troubleshooting tips

- It is essential to image the lower pole of each kidney because free abdominal fluid also accumulates in this area.

- If the image generated during an eFAST exam is suboptimal, the examination is non-diagnostic. Do not make clinical decisions based on suboptimal images.

- If the subxiphoid view of the heart is unavailable due to abdominal pain, use other ultrasound views of the heart.

- Ultrasound examination of the pelvis is easier when the bladder is full.

Case closed:

The **25** year-old trauma patient is found to have free fluid in Morison's pouch and the spleno-renal space on ultrasound examination. She is presumed to have intra-abdominal bleeding secondary to trauma. As volume expanders are administered, a trauma surgeon is consulted.

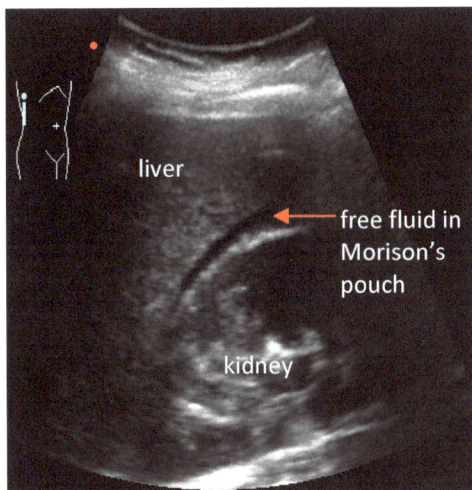

Free fluid in Morison's pouch.

7. Abdominal aortic aneurysm

Case scenario:

A **70 year-old man** presents himself to the clinic complaining of abdominal pain that is radiating to his back. His only medication is an ACE inhibitor for hypertension. His heart rate is **100 beats per minute,** his blood pressure is **90/40 mmHg,** and he appears to be in distress. Due to his obesity, it is difficult to palpate deep abdominal structures on a physical exam.

Impression: Abdominal pain NYD, rule out an abdominal aortic aneurysm.

An abdominal aortic aneurysm (AAA) is a localized dilation of the abdominal aorta. This chapter will review the technique for imaging the abdominal aorta with bedside ultrasound and illustrate how to recognize an AAA.

7.1. Probe choice

To image the abdominal aorta, use a low frequency curvilinear probe or a phased array probe in the abdominal setting. Low frequency probes provide the depth penetration needed to image deep structures like the abdominal aorta.

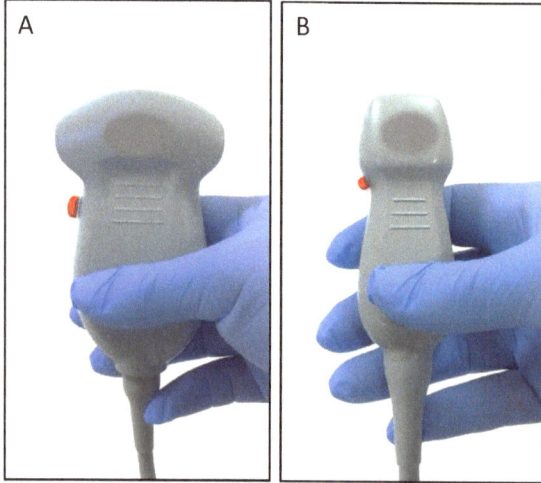

Figure 7.1 Low frequency probes that can be used to assess a patient with a suspected abdominal aortic aneurysm (AAA).

A. A curvilinear probe.
B. A phased array probe. Red circle denotes orientation marker.

7.2. Patient positioning and scanning technique

The patient should be in the supine position, with the knees slightly bent to relax the abdominal musculature. Start in the epigastric area with the probe held in the transverse plane. The orientation marker should point to the patient's right. Identify the abdominal aorta first and then scan in the transverse plane every centimeter down to the bifurcation of the aorta into the iliac arteries (Noble et al., 2007; Reardon et al., 2008).

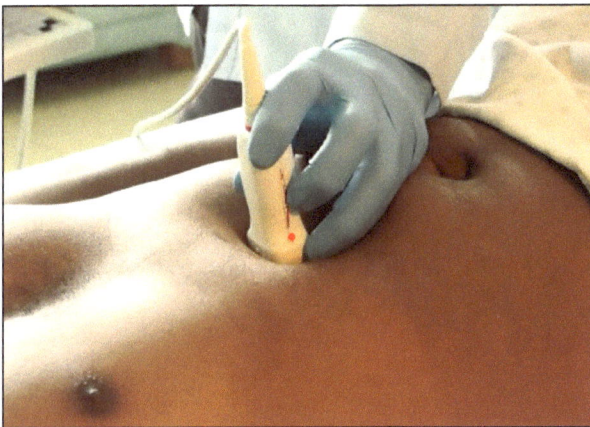

Video 7.1 Scanning technique for imaging the abdominal aorta in the transverse plane.

Red circle denotes orientation marker. View video online at bedsideultrasoundlevel1.com

An important landmark to identify on the ultrasound image is the **vertebral body.** The anterior aspect of the vertebral body appears as a hyperechoic (white) structure. The vertebral body casts a shadow deep to its hyperechoic surface because ultrasound cannot penetrate bone. The abdominal aorta appears as a round anechoic (black) structure, anterior and to the right of the vertebral body on the ultrasound monitor.

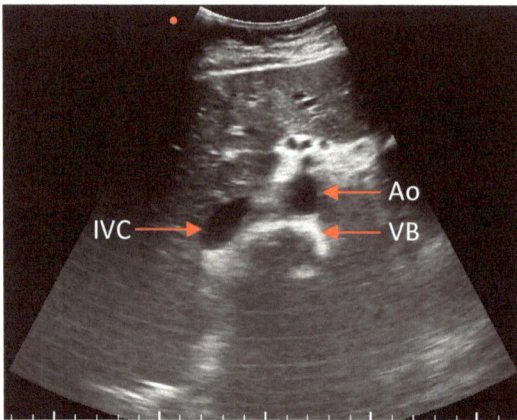

Figure 7.2 The abdominal aorta in the transverse plane.

The aorta (Ao) is anterior and to the right of the vertebral body (VB). The inferior vena cava (IVC) is also anterior but to the left of the vertebral body. Red circle denotes orientation marker.

Table 7.1 Characteristics of the ultrasound image used to differentiate the abdominal aorta from the inferior vena cava (IVC).

Characteristics	Abdominal aorta	IVC
Shape	Round	Tear-shaped
Walls	Thick	Thin
Respiratory variability in diameter	No	Yes
Position relative to vertebral body	Anterior and screen-right	Anterior and screen-left

The aorta should also be visualized in the sagittal plane. First locate the vessel in the transverse plane, then rotate the probe clockwise 90°. The aorta is now imaged in the sagittal plane. The proximal aorta will be on screen left, the distal aorta on screen right.

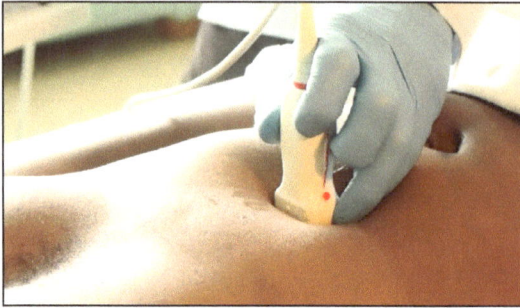

Video 7.2 Scanning technique for imaging the abdominal aorta in the sagittal plane with a phased array probe.

Red circle denotes orientation marker. View video online at bedsideultrasoundlevel1.com

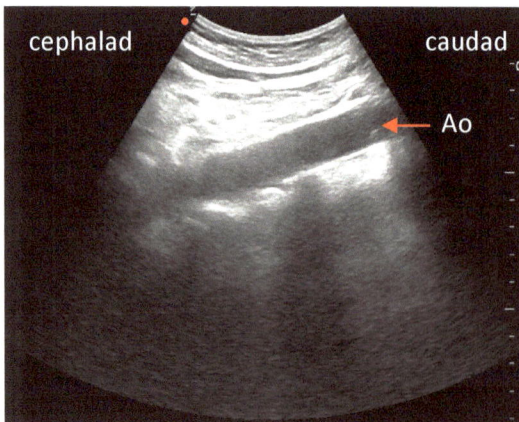

Figure 7.3 The abdominal aorta in the sagittal plane.

Ao: Aorta. Red circle denotes orientation marker.

7.3. Clinical relevance - Abdominal aortic aneurysm

An AAA is present when the diameter of the aorta is greater than 3 cm. The anteroposterior diameter of the aorta should be measured from outer wall to outer wall in both the transverse and sagittal plane (Middleton et al., 2004; Noble et al., 2007; Reardon et al., 2008). Bedside ultrasound is accurate in diagnosing an AAA (Tayal et al., 2003). However, it is insensitive in identifying the presence of retroperitoneal blood associated with a ruptured AAA (Shuman et al., 1988).

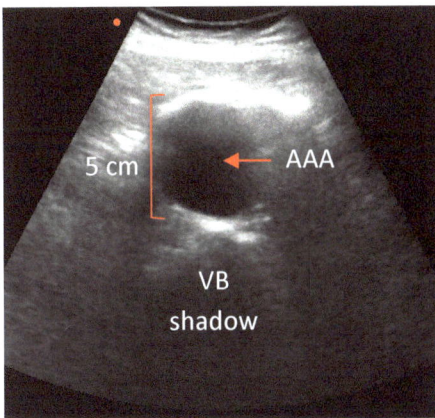

Figure 7.4 An abdominal aortic aneurysm (AAA) in the transverse plane.

The diameter of the aorta is greater than 3 cm from outer wall to outer wall. VB: vertebral body. Red circle denotes orientation marker.

An intraluminal clot within an AAA may falsely suggest a normal aortic diameter. This is because the edge of the clot may be mistaken for the aortic wall.

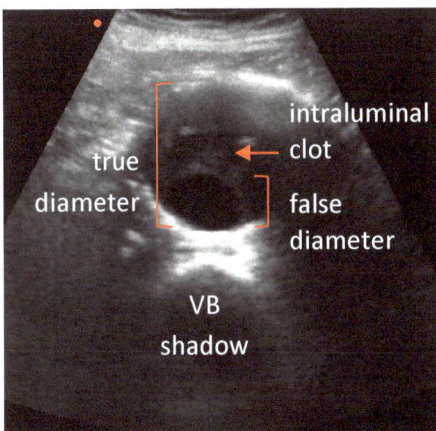

Figure 7.5 An abdominal aortic aneurysm (AAA) with intraluminal clot.

The true diameter of the AAA is 7 cm. VB: vertebral body. Red circle denotes orientation marker.

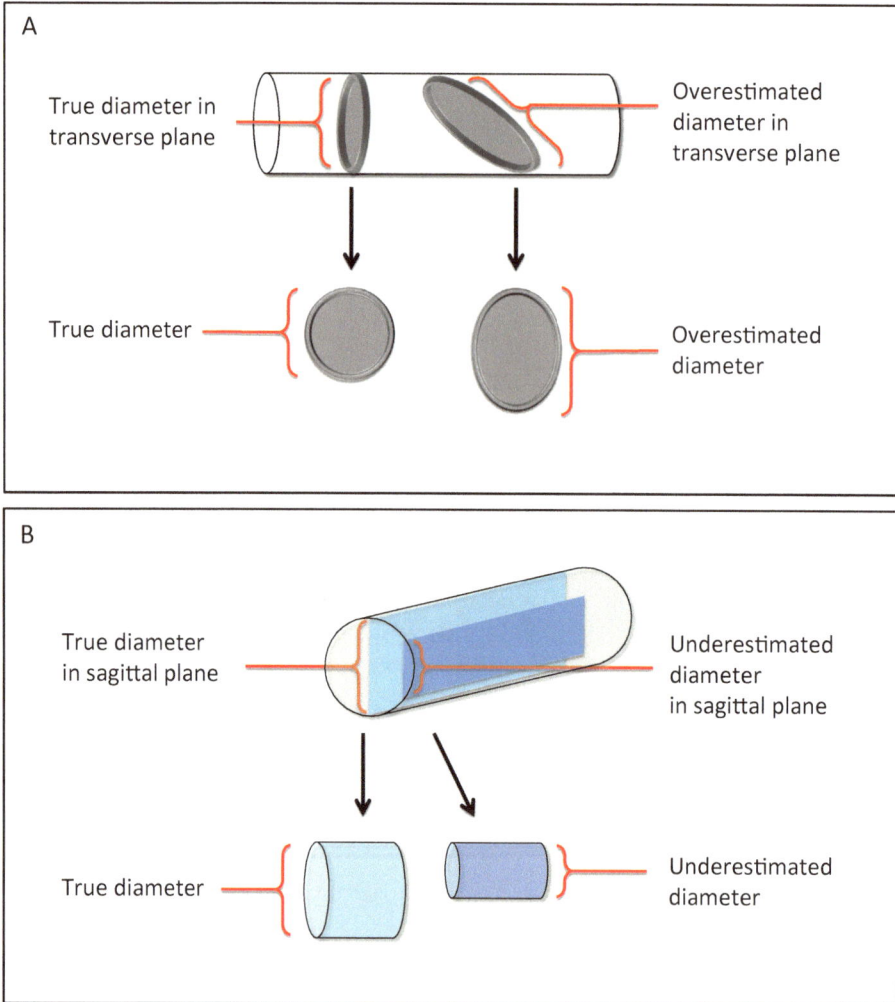

Figure 7.6 Estimating the true aortic diameter in the transverse and sagittal plane.

A. Estimating the aortic diameter in the transverse plane must be performed with the plane of view perpendicular to the vessel.
B. Estimating the aortic diameter in the sagittal plane must be performed with the plane of view at the center of the vessel.

7.4. Troubleshooting tips

- Bleeding from the aorta is usually retroperitoneal and difficult to identify with ultrasound.

- Bowel gas sometimes obscures the image of the abdominal aorta. To move the bowel out of the way, apply gentle pressure on the abdomen with the probe. Asking the patient to take a large breath may also move the bowel out of the way.

- In obese patients, the abdominal aorta may be difficult to image. Image generation can be facilitated by:

  ➢ Placing patients in the left or right lateral decubitus position.

  ➢ Lowering the frequency of the probe to increase penetration of the ultrasound beam.

Case closed:

The 70 year-old man is found to have a large 5 cm AAA on ultrasound examination. The AAA was visualized upon placing the patient in the right lateral decubitus position. A vascular surgeon is urgently consulted.

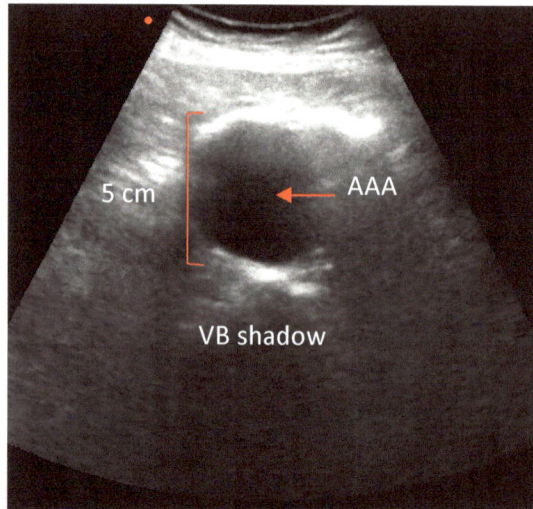

An abdominal aortic aneurysm (AAA) in the transverse plane.

8. Cholecystitis

Case scenario:

A 60 year-old obese man with no significant past medical history presents himself to the clinic with postprandial abdominal pain. Examination reveals a man with a fever of 38.5°C, otherwise normal vital signs, and right upper quadrant tenderness on palpation.

Impression: Abdominal pain, must rule out cholecystitis.

Cholecystitis is an inflammation of the gallbladder often caused by the obstruction of the cystic duct by gallstones. This chapter will review the technique for imaging the gallbladder with bedside ultrasound, and illustrate the basic ultrasonographic signs of cholecystitis.

8.1. Probe choice

To image the gallbladder, use a low frequency curvilinear probe or a phased array probe in the abdominal setting. Low frequency probes provide the depth penetration necessary to image deep structures like the gallbladder.

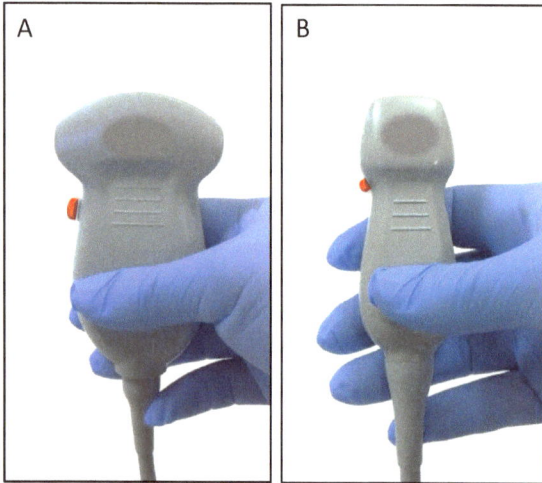

Figure 8.1 Low frequency probes that can be used to assess a patient with suspected cholecystitis.
A. A curvilinear probe.
B. A phased array probe. Red circle denotes orientation marker.

8.2. Patient position and scanning technique

There are three basic techniques to image the gallbladder in a supine patient:

Technique #1: The subcostal sweep

Technique #2: The X-7 approach

Technique #3: The posterolateral approach

Technique #1: The subcostal sweep

The patient lies in the supine position with knees slightly bent in order to relax the abdominal muscles. The probe is held in the sagittal plane with the orientation marker pointing cephalad. Place the probe below the costal margin in the epigastric area and sweep along the right costal margin laterally.

In general, the gallbladder will come into view in the right subcostal area at the mid-clavicular line. Since the gallbladder is generally under the ribs, the probe must be pointing slightly cephalad.

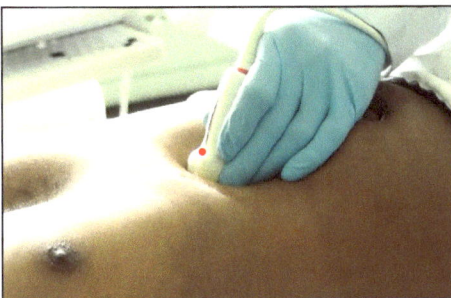

Video 8.1 Scanning Technique #1: The subcostal sweep for imaging the gallbladder.

The gallbladder is generally found in the mid-clavicular line. Red circle denotes orientation marker. View video online at bedsideultrasoundlevel1.com

97

Technique #2: The X-7 approach

The 'X' refers to the xiphoid region. The probe is placed 7 cm lateral and to the right of the xiphoid. The probe is held in the transverse plane with the orientation marker pointing towards the patient's right. The probe angle must be adjusted such that the ultrasound beam penetrates the intercostal space and avoids the ribs. The gallbladder will often be found at this location.

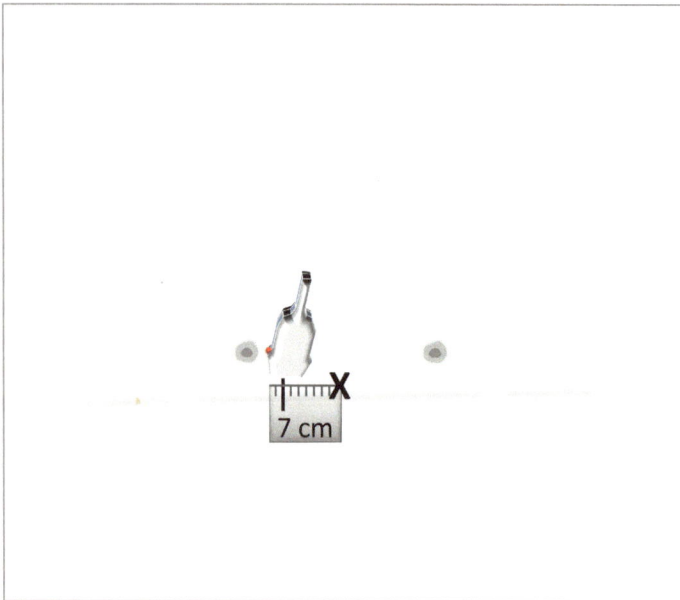

Figure 8.2 Scanning Technique #2: The X-7 technique for imaging the gallbladder.

The probe is placed 7 cm laterally and to the right of the xiphoid (X). Red circle denotes orientation marker.

Technique #3: The posterolateral approach

The probe is placed over the right posterolateral flank with the orientation marker pointing cephalad. Once Morison's pouch has been identified (the potential space between the liver and the upper pole of the right kidney; Section 6.3), the probe is moved anteriorly until the gallbladder comes into view.

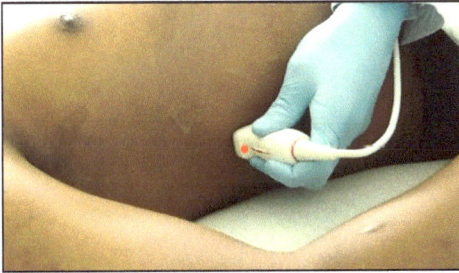

Video 8.2 Scanning Technique #3: The posterolateral approach for imaging the gallbladder.

Red circle denotes orientation marker. View video online at bedsideultrasoundlevel1.com

8.3. Ultrasound appearance of the gallbladder

A normal gallbladder appears as an anechoic (black) structure with thin hyperechoic (white) walls. The gallbladder is surrounded by the hypoechoic (grey) appearing liver. Depending on its position, you may first see the gallbladder in the transverse or longitudinal orientation. A useful landmark to identify the gallbladder in the longitudinal orientation is the **exclamation point sign**. The exclamation point sign is formed by the gallbladder in longitudinal orientation and the portal vein in transverse orientation.

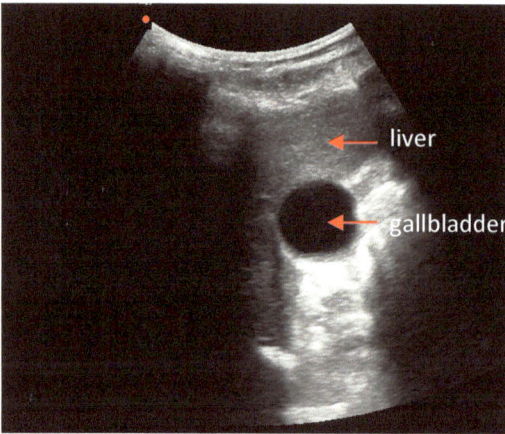

Figure 8.3 The gallbladder imaged in the transverse orientation.

Red circle denotes orientation marker.

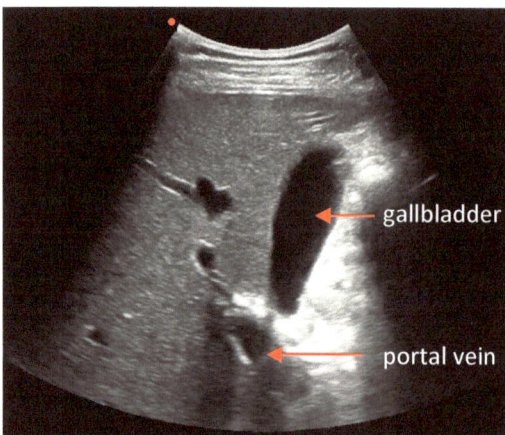

Figure 8.4 The exclamation point sign: gallbladder imaged in the longitudinal orientation.

The exclamation point sign is formed by the gallbladder in longitudinal orientation and the portal vein in transverse orientation. Red circle denotes orientation marker.

It is important to scan through the gallbladder in **both the transverse and the longitudinal orientation**. First sweep through the gallbladder from the fundus to the neck in the transverse orientation. Then turn the probe 90°, find the gallbladder in the longitudinal orientation, and sweep through from side-to-side.

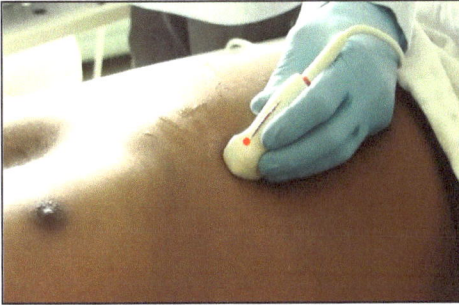

Video 8.3 Scanning technique for imaging the gallbladder in the longitudinal and transverse orientation using a phased array probe.

Red circle denotes orientation marker. View video online at bedsideultrasoundlevel1.com

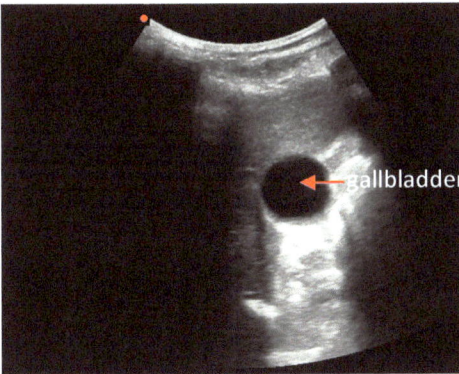

Video 8.4 The gallbladder being imaged in the transverse orientation from the fundus to the neck.

Red circle denotes orientation marker. View video online at bedsideultrasoundlevel1.com

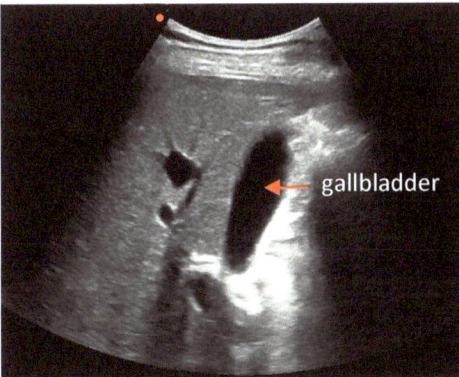

Video 8.5 The gallbladder being imaged in the longitudinal orientation from side-to-side.

Red circle denotes orientation marker. View video online at bedsideultrasoundlevel1.com

8.4. Clinical relevance: Cholecystitis

Cholecystitis is often caused by the obstruction of the cystic duct by gallstones. Three important ultrasonographic signs to look for in diagnosing cholecystitis are:

        Sign #1: Gallstones

        Sign #2: Sonographic Murphy sign

        Sign #3: Thickness of anterior gallbladder wall

Sign #1. Gallstones

Stones within the gallbladder are referred to as either **cholelithiasis** or **gallstones**. Gallstones appear hyperechoic (white) and cast a shadow into the far-field of the ultrasound image. The presence of a shadow differentiates gallstones from structures that do not cast a shadow such as gallbladder polyps, tumors, or thickened bile (sludge).

Most gallstones are mobile, and lie on the dependent side of the gallbladder. Therefore, this characteristic can be useful in identifying a gallstone - if the patient changes position, the gallstone will move and settle to the dependent side of the gallbladder. However, there are two exceptions to this rule:

- Cholesterol gallstones float and so do not settle to the dependent side of the gallbladder

- Gallstones that are impacted in the neck of the gallbladder will not move as the patient changes position

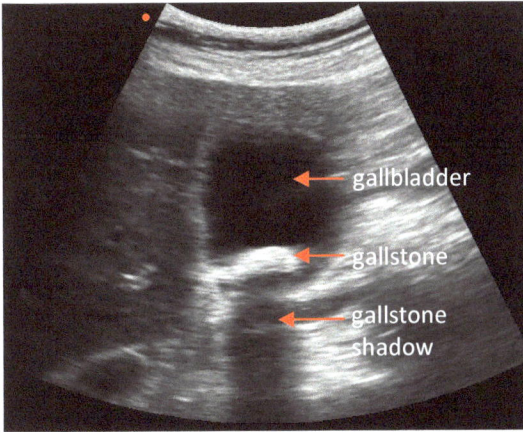

Figure 8.5 The gallbladder in transverse orientation showing a gallstone.

Gallstones appear as hyperechoic (white) structures within the gallbladder lumen. They cast a dark shadow into the far-field of the ultrasound screen. Red circle denotes orientation marker.

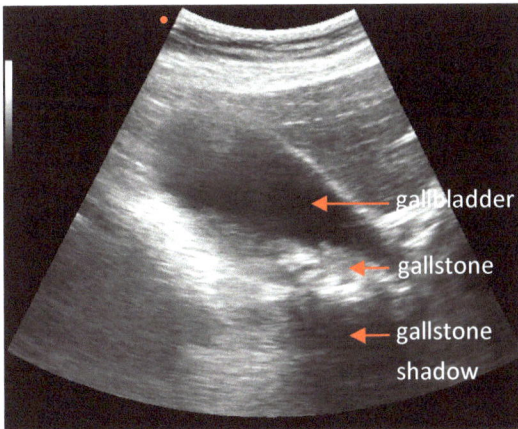

Figure 8.6 The gallbladder in the longitudinal orientation showing gallstones at the neck of the gallbladder.

The gallstones cast a shadow. Red circle denotes orientation marker.

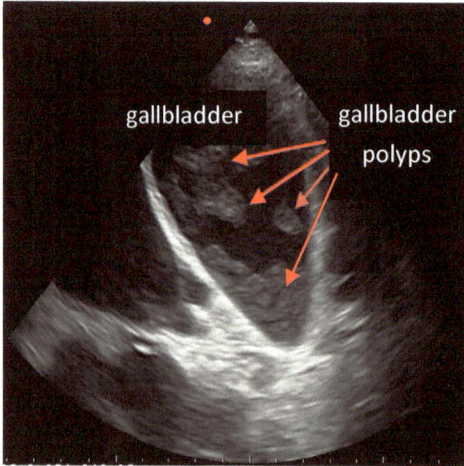

Figure 8.7 The gallbladder in the longitudinal orientation showing multiple gallbladder polyps.

Gallbladder polyps do not cast shadows. Red circle denotes orientation marker.

Sign #2. Sonographic Murphy sign

To elicit a sonographic Murphy sign, use the subcostal approach. The probe is placed just below the ribs so that it is close to the gallbladder. As the patient breathes in, the gallbladder descends and pushes against the probe tip. A positive sonographic Murphy sign is when the patient stops breathing due to pain ("inspiratory arrest").

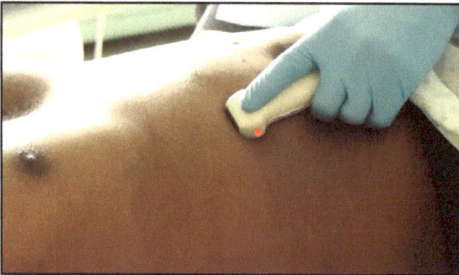

Video 8.6 Scanning technique to elicit a positive sonographic Murphy sign with a phased array probe.

Red circle denotes orientation marker. View video online at bedsideultrasoundlevel1.com

Sign #3. Thickness of anterior gallbladder wall

The anterior (near-field) gallbladder wall is commonly measured in the transverse orientation. The anterior wall is <3 mm in thickness in a normal gallbladder.

The posterior (far-field) gallbladder wall will appear thickened due to acoustic enhancement and is thus not used for measuring wall thickness.

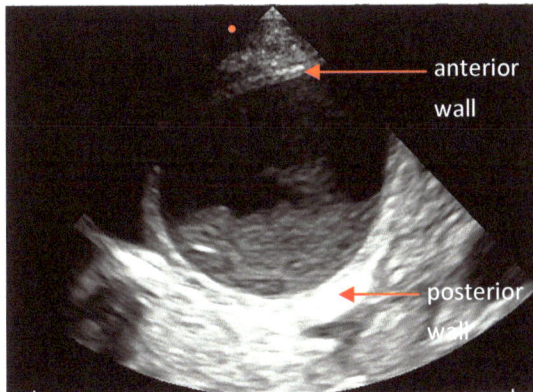

Figure 8.8 Anterior and posterior wall of the gallbladder.
Red circle denotes orientation marker.

Thickening of the anterior gallbladder wall >3 mm can be seen in cholecystitis. It is also associated with other conditions (Engel et al., 1980; Finberg et al., 1979):

- Hypoproteinemia
- Cirrhosis
- Congestive heart failure
- Hepatitis
- Renal failure
- Ascites
- Postprandial state

Summary - Clinical relevance for cholecystitis

In a patient with right upper quadrant abdominal pain suspected of having cholecystitis:

- The presence of a positive sonographic Murphy sign has a positive predictive value of 43-72% for cholecystitis (Bree, 1995; Ralls et al., 1982)

- The combination of a positive sonographic Murphy sign and gallstones has a positive predictive value of 92% for cholecystitis (Ralls et al., 1985)

- Gallstones combined with an anterior gallbladder wall thickness greater than 3 mm has a positive predictive value of 95% for cholecystitis (Ralls, Colletti et al., 1985)

8.5. Troubleshooting tips

- In Technique #1 (subcostal sweep), the gallbladder is sometimes better visualized with the patient in the left lateral decubitus position.

- In Technique #1, the gallbladder is generally found in the mid-clavicular line, but can also be found anywhere between the epigastrium and the right mid-axillary line.

- In cases where the gallbladder is difficult to image, having the patient breathe in and hold their breath can descend the gallbladder into the ultrasound field.

- The gallbladder contracts after a patient has eaten, and is thus best visualized in a fasting patient.

- The shadowing caused by air in the duodenum can sometimes be mistaken for a gallstone shadow.

Case closed:

The 60 year-old obese man with postprandial abdominal pain has gallstones and a positive sonographic Murphy sign on ultrasound examination. Cholecystitis is suspected, and he is referred to a surgeon for further care.

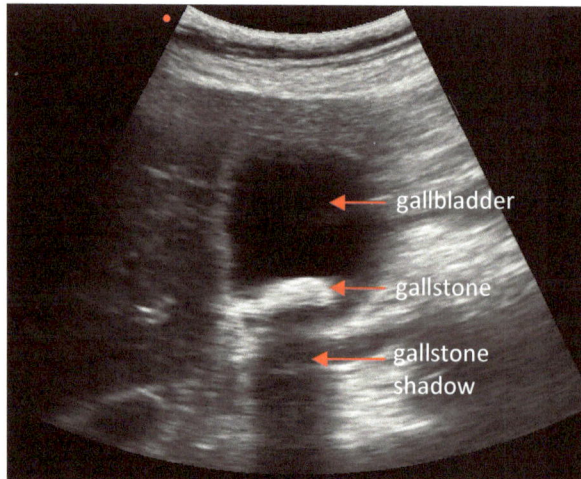

The gallbladder in transverse orientation showing a gallstone.

9. Kidney injury

> **Case scenario:**
>
> **An 80 year-old man presents himself to your office with generalized weakness and dyspnea. He notes decreased urine output over several weeks. On exam, the patient has pitting edema of the lower extremities and a fullness in the suprapubic area. His serum creatinine level was normal six months ago but is now high at 365 μmol/L.**
>
> **Impression: Acute kidney injury, rule out obstructive cause.**

One cause of **kidney injury** is an obstruction to urine flow between the kidney and urethra. This type of kidney injury is called **post-renal failure**, and can be identified using bedside ultrasound (Swadron et al., 2008). This chapter will review the technique for imaging the kidney and bladder, and illustrate how to diagnose post-renal failure.

9.1. Probe choice

In order to image the kidney and bladder, use a low frequency curvilinear probe or a phased array probe in the abdominal setting. Low frequency probes provide the depth penetration needed to image deep structures like the kidney and bladder.

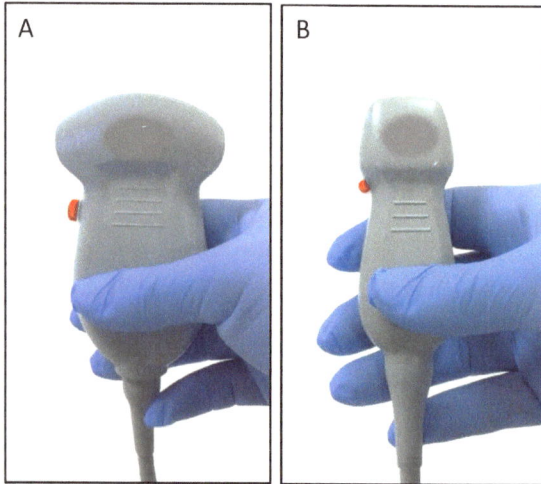

Figure 9.1 Low frequency probes that can be used to assess a patient with kidney injury.

A. A curvilinear probe.
B. A phased array probe. Red circle denotes orientation marker.

9.2. Patient position and scanning technique

Imaging the kidney in the coronal plane

The patient is examined in the supine position. Look for the kidney with the probe in the posterior axillary line approximately level with the xiphoid. The orientation marker on the probe is pointing cephalad and slightly posteriorly.

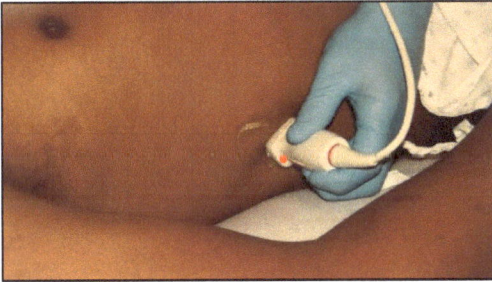

Figure 9.2 Scanning technique for imaging the right kidney in the coronal plane with a phased array probe.

The probe is in the coronal plane with the orientation marker pointing cephalad. Red circle denotes orientation marker.

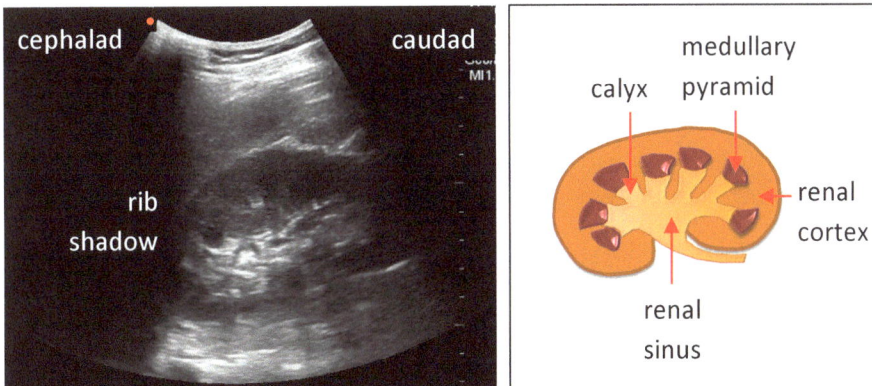

Figure 9.3 The kidney imaged in the coronal plane.

Ultrasound image and corresponding schematic. Red circle denotes orientation marker.

To image the entire kidney in the coronal plane, sweep the ultrasound beam anteroposteriorly.

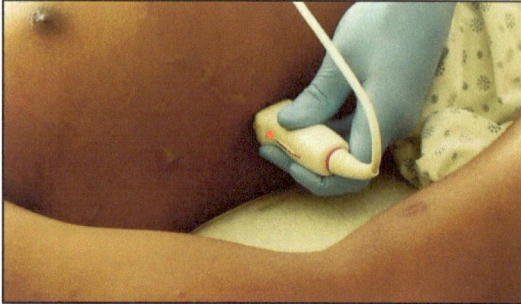

Video 9.1 Scanning technique for imaging the entire kidney in the coronal plane.

Red circle denotes orientation marker. View video online at bedsideultrasoundlevel1.com

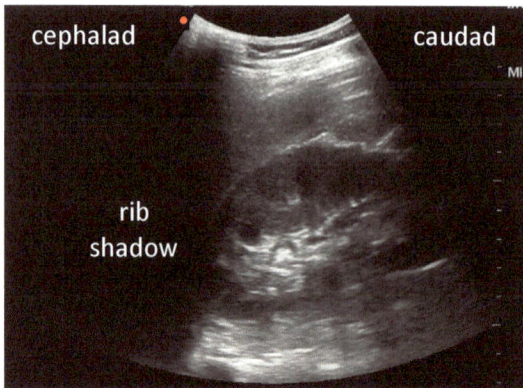

Video 9.2 The kidney imaged in the coronal plane while sweeping the probe anteroposteriorly.

Red circle denotes orientation marker. View video online at bedsideultrasoundlevel1.com

Imaging the kidney in the transverse plane

Once the kidney has been located in the coronal plane, turn the probe clockwise 90°. The orientation marker is now pointing anteriorly. This adjustment provides an image of the kidney in the transverse plane. To image the entire kidney in the transverse plane, sweep the ultrasound beam from upper to lower pole.

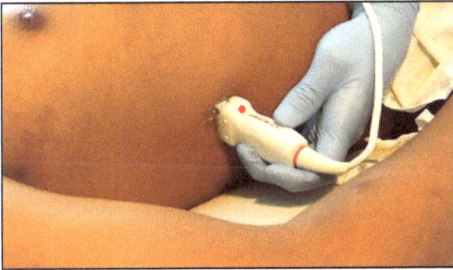

Video 9.3 Scanning technique for imaging the right kidney in the transverse plane from upper to lower pole.

Sweep the probe from cephalad to caudad. Red circle denotes orientation marker. View video online at bedsideultrasoundlevel1.com

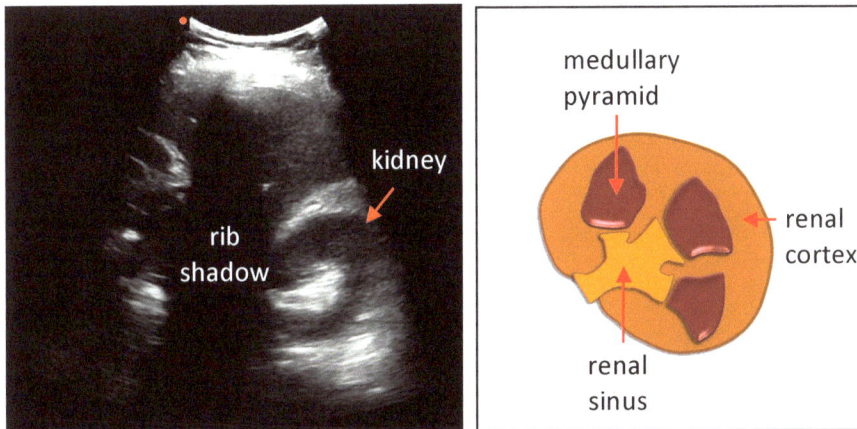

Video 9.4 The kidney imaged in the transverse plane while sweeping the probe from cephalad to caudad.

Ultrasound image and corresponding schematic. Red circle denotes orientation marker. View video online at bedsideultrasoundlevel1.com

Imaging the bladder in the sagittal plane

To image the bladder in the sagittal plane, place the probe just above the symphysis pubis, with the orientation marker pointing cephalad. Angle the probe caudally. The urine in the bladder appears anechoic (black).

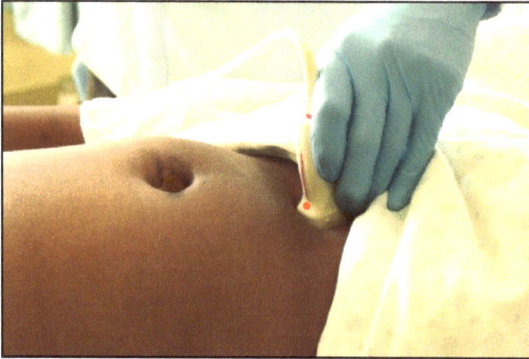

Figure 9.4 Scanning technique for imaging the bladder in the sagittal plane.
Red circle denotes orientation marker.

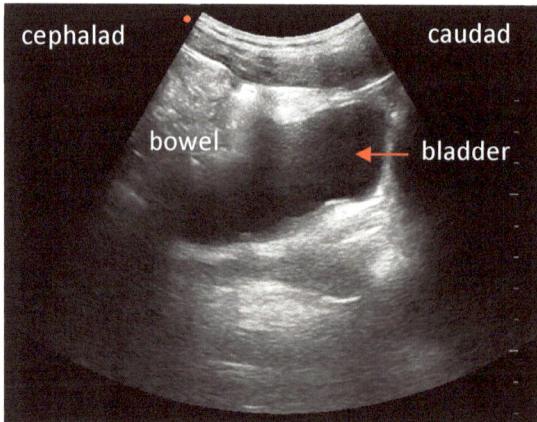

Figure 9.5 The male bladder imaged in the sagittal plane.
Red circle denotes orientation marker.

Imaging the bladder in the transverse plane

To image the bladder in the transverse plane, place the probe just above the symphysis pubis, with the orientation marker pointing to the patient's right. Angle the probe caudally.

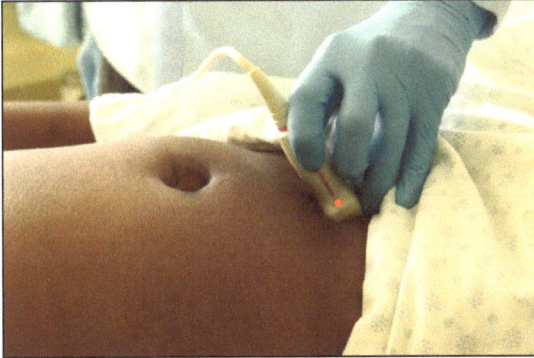

Figure 9.6 Scanning technique for imaging the bladder in the transverse plane.

Red circle denotes orientation marker.

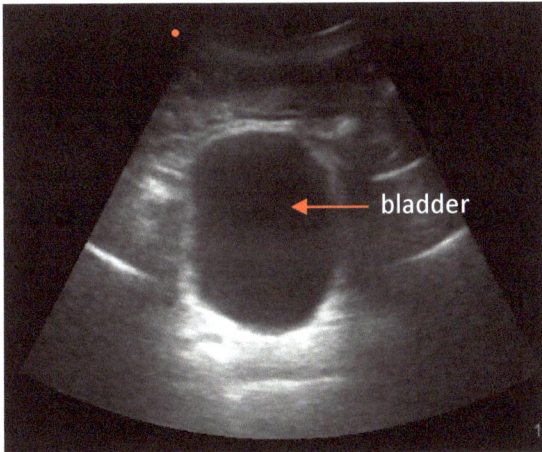

Figure 9.7 The male bladder in the transverse plane.

Red circle denotes orientation marker.

9.3. Clinical relevance - Obstructive causes of kidney injury

Ultrasound is useful in identifying obstructive causes of kidney injury (post-renal failure). Hydronephrosis and a distended post-void bladder are ultasonographic signs of obstruction to urinary flow.

Hydronephrosis

Hydronephrosis is a distension of the renal sinus and calyces due to an obstruction of the urinary tract distal to the kidney (Byrne et al., 2013).

Unilateral hydronephrosis is generally due to pathology of the ureter or ureterovesicular junction (e.g. nephrolithiasis).

Bilateral hydronephrosis is generally due to pathology at the level of the bladder (e.g. bladder tumor, neurogenic bladder) or distal to the bladder (e.g. prostatic disease).

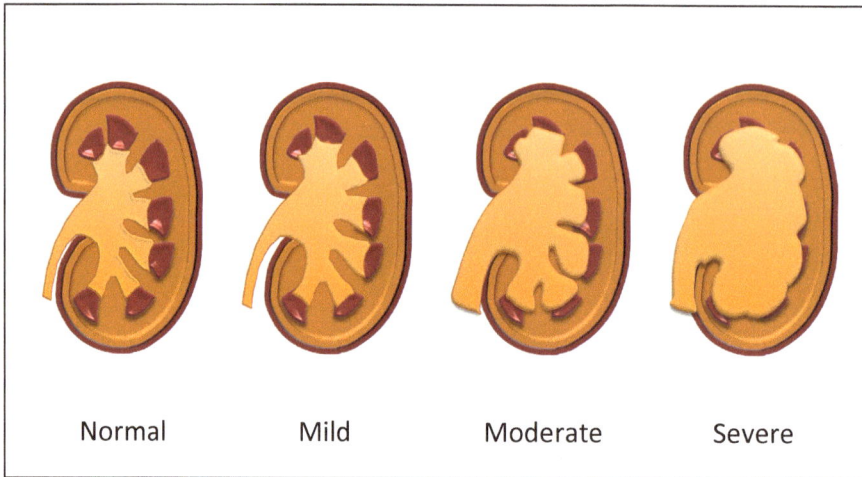

| Normal | Mild | Moderate | Severe |

Figure 9.8 Schematic depicting grades of hydronephrosis.

Mild: *Distension of renal sinus and calyces (collecting system).*
Moderate: *Increased distension of the collecting system.*
Severe: *Ballooning of calyces with cortical thinning.*

In hydronephrosis, the calyces and renal sinus appear anechoic (black) and distended on the ultrasound image.

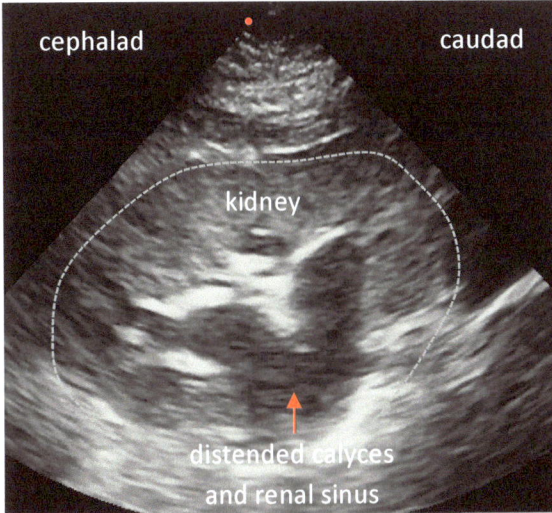

Figure 9.9 The kidney in the coronal plane with moderate hydronephrosis, i.e. "the bear paw sign".

Red circle denotes orientation marker.

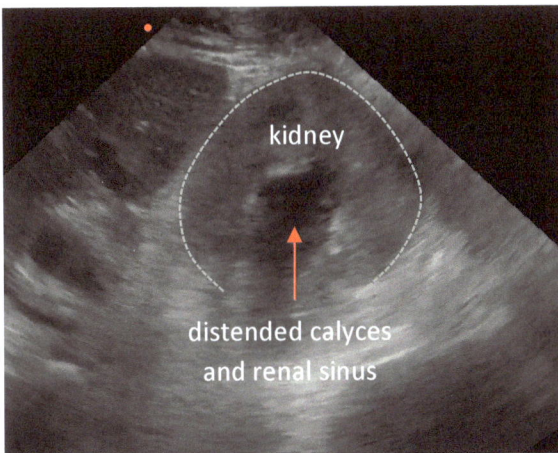

Figure 9.10 The kidney in the transverse plane with moderate hydronephrosis.

Red circle denotes orientation marker.

Distended post-void bladder

The upper limit of normal **post-void bladder volume** is 50-100 ml in an adult patient (Kelly, 2004). However, in patients with chronic incomplete emptying of the bladder, this value can be much higher without associated kidney injury.

Although many portable ultrasound machines have a pre-programmed formula for calculating bladder volume, a gross estimate of post-void bladder volume can be determined using the following formula (Chan, 1993).

$$\text{Bladder volume (ml)} = 0.75 \times (W_{trans} \times H_{trans} \times L_{sagit})$$

W_{trans} = maximum width in transverse plane (cm)

H_{trans} = maximum height in transverse plane (cm)

L_{sagit} = maximum length in sagittal plane (cm)

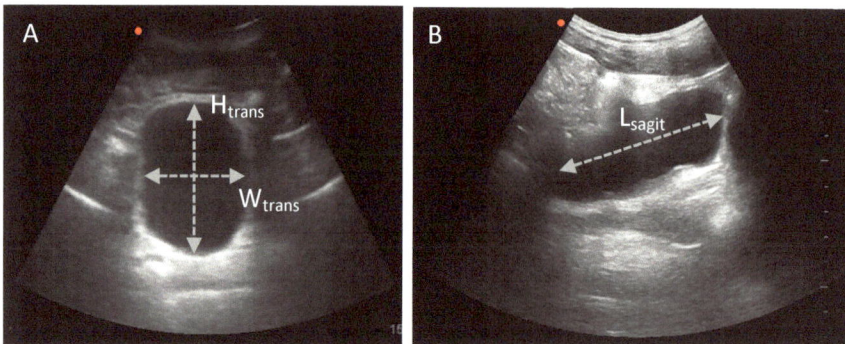

Figure 9.11 Gross estimation of bladder volume.
A. Maximum bladder height and width in transverse plane.
B. Maximum bladder length in sagittal plane. Red circle denotes orientation marker.

The assessment of post-void bladder volume is clinically relevant in the following common scenarios:

- A patient presents with kidney injury and is found to have a high post-void residual bladder volume. In an older male patient, this condition is commonly due to prostatic disease

- A patient with a **Foley catheter** stops urinating. If there is a full bladder on ultrasound then the diagnosis is a blocked or misplaced Foley catheter

Table 9.1 Combined kidney and bladder ultrasound findings, and common associated pathologies.

| | Post-void bladder ||
	Full	**Empty**
Hydronephrosis	Pathology at the level of the bladder: • neurogenic bladder • medications Pathology distal to the bladder: • prostatic disease • blocked Foley	Pathology between kidney and UV junction: • bladder tumor • nephrolithiasis • ureteral tumor

9.4. Troubleshooting tips

- **When rib shadows obscure the view of the kidney, ask the patient to breathe in and hold their breath. This action will cause the kidney to descend below the ribs, improving the quality of the image (*see Video 9.5*).**

- **To avoid rib shadows entirely, turn the probe obliquely (upper part of probe angled posteriorly) so the ultrasound beam runs along the intercostal space.**

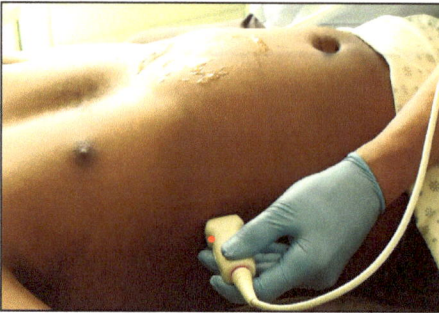

Video 9.5 Scanning technique for removing rib shadows.

Red circle denotes orientation marker. View video online at bedsideultrasoundlevel1.com

Case closed:

The 80 year-old man with acute kidney injury has bilateral hydronephrosis and a full post-void bladder on ultrasound examination. Bladder outlet obstruction is suspected, a Foley catheter is placed, and an urologist is consulted.

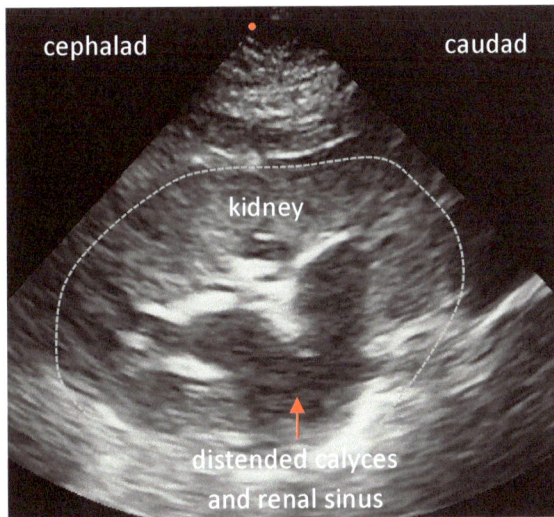

The kidney in the coronal plane with moderate hydronephrosis.

10. Deep venous thrombosis of the lower limb

Case scenario:

A 40 year-old woman with no significant past medical history presents herself to the emergency room with a swollen leg. Her only current medication is the birth control pill. She has just completed a 14 hour flight. Physical exam reveals a swollen, non-tender left leg, no cord, and negative Homan's sign.

Impression: Swollen leg, high suspicion for deep venous thrombosis (DVT).

Traditionally, a complete lower limb venous ultrasound examination with color Doppler and compression is used for the detection of deep venous thrombosis (DVT). In this chapter, we introduce an abbreviated lower limb ultrasound examination using **compression ultrasound** only. The abbreviated examination includes imaging the common femoral vein and the popliteal vein. There is evidence to suggest that an abbreviated compression ultrasound examination of the leg is sufficiently sensitive to detect the majority of clinically significant DVTs of the lower limb in ambulatory patients (Birdwell et al., 1998; Blaivas et al., 2000; Magazzini et al., 2007; Poppiti et al., 1995; Theodoro et al., 2004).

10.1. Probe choice

A high frequency linear probe is used when examining veins. High frequency probes give excellent resolution of superficial structures.

In obese patients or patients with muscular legs, the vascular structures may be too deep to visualize with a high frequency probe. In these cases, a low frequency curvilinear probe can be used.

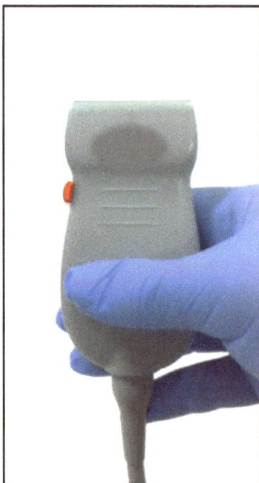

Figure 10.1 A high frequency linear probe is used to assess veins of the lower leg.

Red circle denotes orientation marker.

10.2. Patient position and scanning technique - Common femoral vein

Patients can be evaluated in the supine position with the head of the bed elevated to 30°, thus ensuring engorgement of the lower extremity veins. The leg should be externally rotated with the knee slightly bent.

The probe is placed just below the inguinal ligament with the orientation marker pointing towards the patient's right. This probe position will provide a transverse view of the common femoral vein. Veins appear anechoic (black) on the ultrasound image.

Scan the common femoral vein from the inguinal ligament caudally until the junction between the common femoral vein, femoral vein, and deep femoral vein.

Clinical relevance - DVT in the common femoral vein

During compression ultrasound, the examiner compresses the vein with the ultrasound probe. If the opposing walls of the vein touch each other, a venous thrombosis is excluded at that discrete point. If a DVT is present, the opposing walls of the vein will not touch each other when the vein is compressed. A DVT can also be detected as a slightly hyperechoic (white) structure within the vein lumen (Labropoulos et al., 2005).

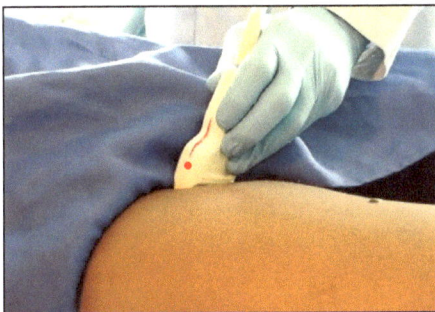

Video 10.1 Scanning technique for compression ultrasound of the common femoral vein.

Red circle denotes orientation marker. View video online at bedsideultrasoundlevel1.com

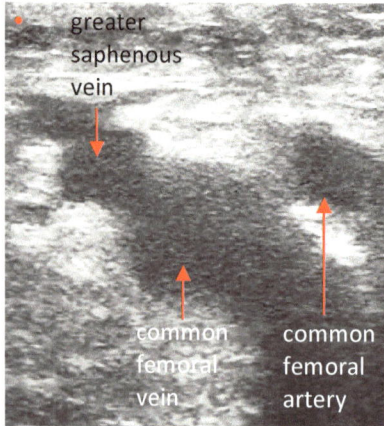

greater
saphenous
vein

common
femoral
vein

common
femoral
artery

Video 10.2 Compression ultrasound of a normal left common femoral vein.

When the vein is compressed, the opposite walls of the vein touch each other, therefore excluding a DVT at this point. Red circle denotes orientation marker. View video online at bedsideultrasoundlevel1.com

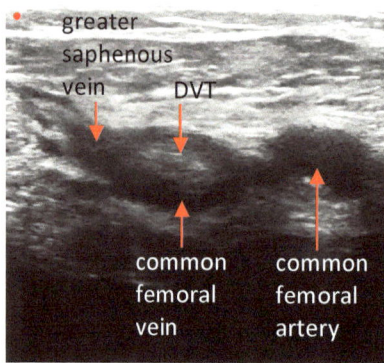

greater
saphenous
vein

DVT

common
femoral
vein

common
femoral
artery

Video 10.3 Compression ultrasound demonstrating a DVT in the left common femoral vein.

When the vein is compressed, the walls of the vein remain separated due to the presence of the DVT. The DVT is hyperechoic (white) and is seen within the lumen of the vein. Red circle denotes orientation marker. View video online at bedsideultrasoundlevel1.com

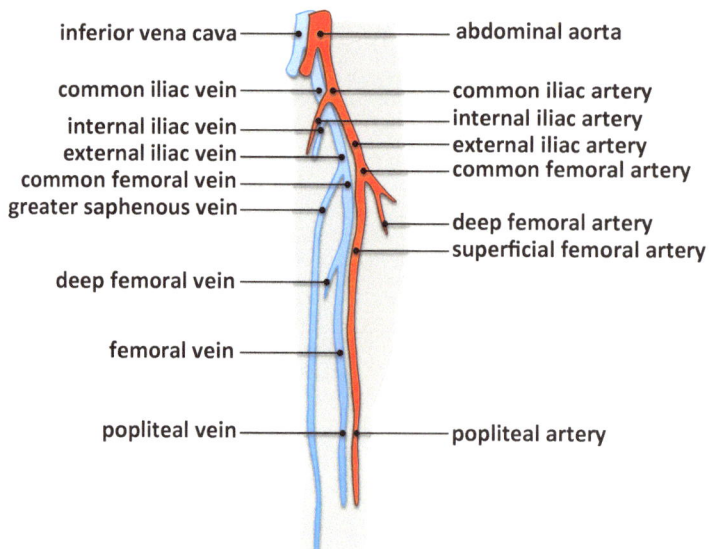

inferior vena cava — abdominal aorta

common iliac vein — common iliac artery

internal iliac vein — internal iliac artery

external iliac vein — external iliac artery

common femoral vein — common femoral artery

greater saphenous vein

deep femoral artery

superficial femoral artery

deep femoral vein

femoral vein

popliteal vein — popliteal artery

Figure 10.2 Schematic of veins and arteries of the upper leg.

There are usually four anatomical patterns observed when ultrasound is performed in the transverse plane between the inguinal ligament and the junction between the common femoral, femoral, and deep femoral veins.

Table 10.1 Anatomical patterns observed from transverse ultrasound examination of the common femoral vein in the caudal direction.

Patterns observed from examination of the common femoral vein		
Pattern 1	Junction of the greater saphenous vein (GSV) with the common femoral vein (CFV). The common femoral artery (CFA) is lateral to the CFV	medial lateral GSV CFV CFA
Pattern 2	Common femoral vein (CFV) medial to bifurcation of the common femoral artery into the superficial (SFA) and deep femoral arteries (DFA)	SFA CFV DFA
Pattern 3	The femoral vein (FV) and deep femoral vein (DFV) medial to superficial artery (SFA)	SFA FV DFV
Pattern 4	The femoral vein (FV) posterior to the superficial femoral artery (SFA)	SFA FV

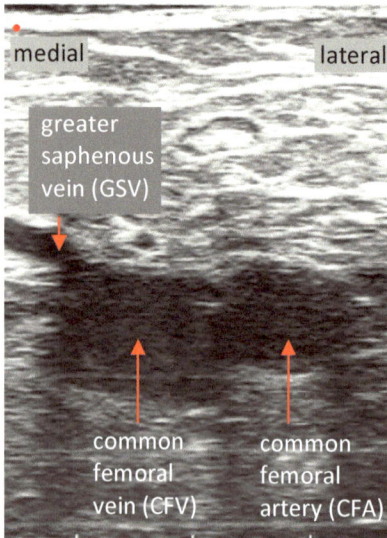

Figure 10.3 Pattern 1: Junction of the greater saphenous vein with the left common femoral vein.

This pattern is seen immediately caudal to the inguinal ligament. The greater saphenous vein enters the common femoral vein medially. The common femoral artery is lateral to the common femoral vein. Red circle denotes orientation marker.

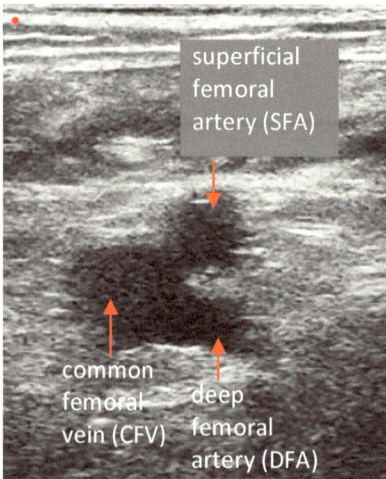

Figure 10.4 Pattern 2: Common femoral vein medial to bifurcation of femoral artery.

The common femoral artery bifurcates several centimeters caudal to Pattern 1. Red circle denotes orientation marker.

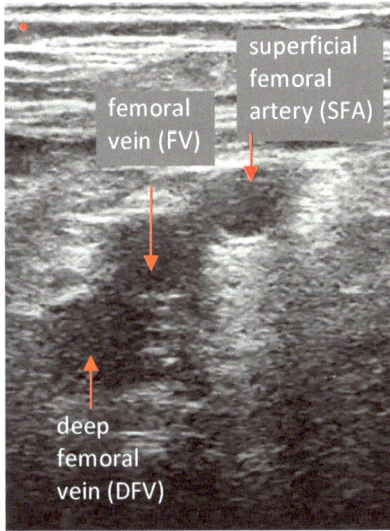

Figure 10.5 Pattern 3: The femoral vein and deep femoral vein medial to the superficial femoral artery.

The deep femoral artery is no longer visible. Red circle denotes orientation marker.

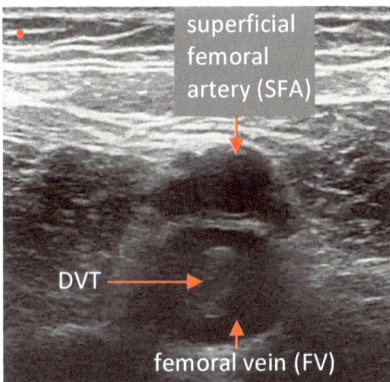

Figure 10.6 Pattern 4: The femoral vein posterior to the superficial femoral artery.

The deep femoral vein is no longer visible. The hyperechoic (white) structure within the femoral vein is a DVT. Red circle denotes orientation marker.

Once compression ultrasound has been completed distally to the junction between the common femoral, femoral, and deep femoral veins, leave the upper leg and proceed to examine the popliteal vein on the same leg (see next section).

10.3. Patient position and scanning technique - Popliteal vein

The popliteal vein can be examined with the patient lying in the supine position, the hips externally rotated, and knees slightly bent. The head of the bed is elevated to 30° to ensure the leg veins are engorged with blood. The orientation marker on the probe faces the patient's right, providing a transverse image of the popliteal vein.

Compression ultrasound of the popliteal vein is performed at every centimeter from the proximal popliteal fossa until the calf. The popliteal vein is superficial to the popliteal artery.

The examination of the popliteal vein is complete when the calf has been reached. At the calf, the popliteal vein divides into the anterior tibial and the tibioperoneal trunk.

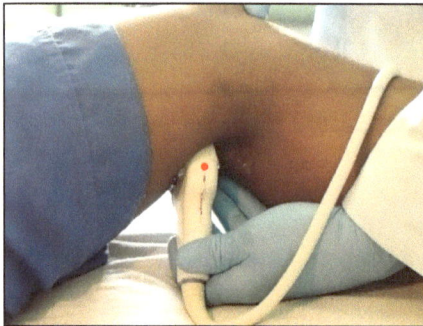

Video 10.4 Scanning technique for compression ultrasound of the popliteal vein.

Red circle denotes orientation marker. View video online at bedsideultrasoundlevel1.com

Clinical relevance - DVT in the popliteal vein

During compression ultrasound of the popliteal vein, the examiner compresses the vein with the ultrasound probe. If the opposing walls of the vein touch each other, a venous thrombosis is excluded at that discrete point. If a DVT is present, the opposing walls of the vein will not touch each other when the vein is compressed.

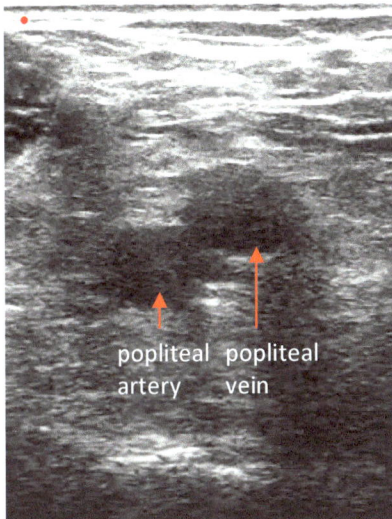

popliteal artery   popliteal vein

Video 10.5 Compression ultrasound of a normal popliteal vein.

The popliteal vein collapses when compressed, excluding a DVT at this point. The artery does not collapse when compressed. Red circle denotes orientation marker. View video online at bedsideultrasoundlevel1.com

10.4. Troubleshooting tips

- To better visualize the popliteal vein, the patient may be examined while sitting or in a prone position.

- Anatomic variance: There may be two popliteal veins in the same leg.

- In obese patients with swollen legs, lowering the frequency of the probe increases depth penetration and may improve the quality of the image.

- The femoral vein is sometimes referred to as the superficial femoral vein. This can be confusing as a thrombus in this vein is considered a DVT.

Case closed:

The 40 year-old woman with a swollen leg has a hyperechoic (white) structure within the common femoral vein on ultrasound examination. The vein does not collapse completely on compression ultrasound, suggesting a DVT. Appropriate anti-coagulation is ordered.

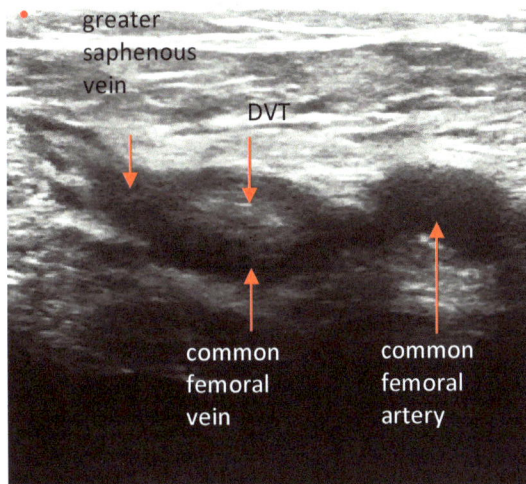

A DVT within the lumen of the left common femoral vein.

11. Ectopic pregnancy

Case scenario:

A 30 year-old woman with a history of pelvic inflammatory disease presents herself to your rural clinic with vaginal bleeding and pelvic pain. Her LMP was seven or eight weeks ago. Her vital signs are stable. A qualitative urinary B HCG test is positive.

Impression: Rule out ectopic pregnancy.

The goal of this chapter is to introduce the use of trans-abdominal pelvic ultrasound as an adjunct in the assessment of a patient with a possible ectopic pregnancy.

11.1. Probe choice

In order to image the female pelvis, use a low frequency curvilinear probe or a phased array probe in the abdominal setting. Low frequency probes provide the depth penetration needed to image deep structures like the uterus.

Transvaginal ultrasound technique and probes will not be discussed in this introductory book.

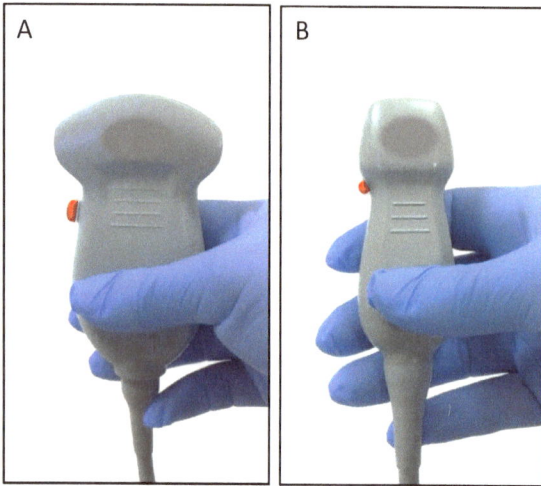

Figure 11.1 Low frequency probes that can be used to assess a patient with suspected ectopic pregnancy.
A. A curvilinear probe.
B. A phased array probe. Red circle denotes orientation marker.

11.2. Patient position and scanning technique

The patient is examined in the supine position with a full bladder.

Imaging the uterus in the transverse plane

The uterus is a mobile organ and thus rarely lies exactly at the midline. To scan the uterus in the transverse plane, place the probe just above the symphysis pubis with the orientation marker pointing to the patient's right. Sweep the probe caudally. To ensure complete imaging of the uterus, scan from the fundus to the cervix in the transverse plane.

The uterus appears as a hypoechoic (grey) round structure below the bladder. An important landmark in the non-pregnant uterus is the **endometrial stripe**. The endometrial stripe is visible at the center of the uterus.

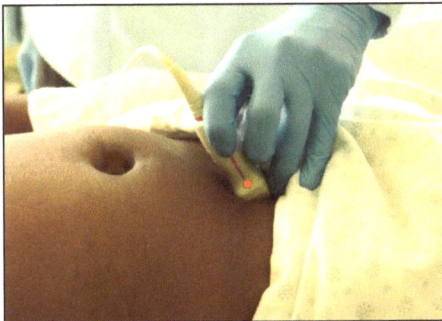

Figure 11.2 Scanning technique for imaging the uterus in the transverse plane using a phased array probe.
Red circle denotes orientation marker.

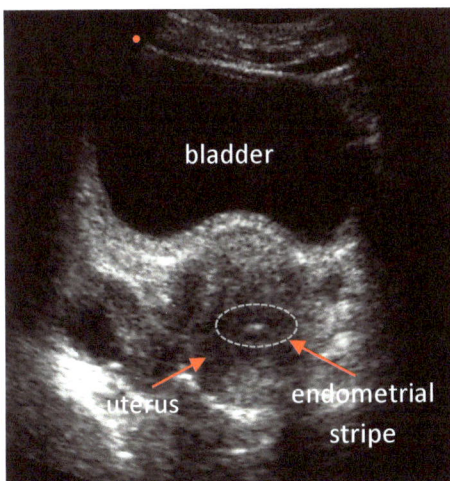

Figure 11.3 The female pelvis imaged in the transverse plane.
Red circle denotes orientation marker.

Imaging the uterus in the sagittal plane

To scan the uterus in the sagittal plane, place the probe just above the symphysis pubis with the orientation marker pointing cephalad. Sweep the probe caudally. To ensure complete imaging of the uterus, sweep the probe by 45° to the right and left while in the sagittal plane.

The uterus appears as a hypoechoic (grey) pear-shaped structure below the bladder. The endometrial stripe appears as a hyperechoic (white) line in the center of the uterus.

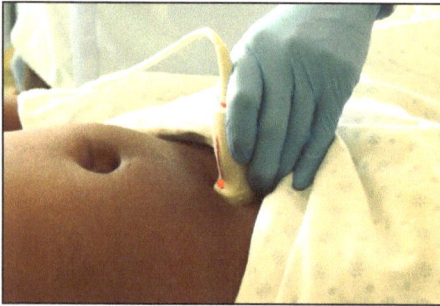

Figure 11.4 Scanning technique for imaging the uterus in the sagittal plane using a phased array probe.
Red circle denotes orientation marker.

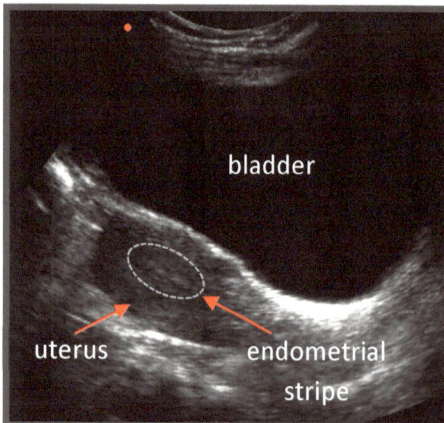

Figure 11.5 The female pelvis imaged in the sagittal plane.
Red circle denotes orientation marker.

138

11.3. The appearance of an intra-uterine pregnancy

There are several signs of first trimester intra-uterine pregnancy on ultrasound examination (Middleton et al., 2004; Noble et al., 2007; Nordenholz et al., 2006; Reardon et al., 2008).

Sign #1: Gestational sac

Sign #2: Yolk sac

Sign #3: Fetal pole

Sign#4: Fetal cardiac activity

The first sign of an intra-uterine pregnancy on the ultrasound image is a **gestational sac**. The gestational sac appears at 5-6 weeks gestational age as an anechoic (black) area within the uterus. The presence of a gestational sac is insufficient for diagnosing an intra-uterine pregnancy because a "pseudogestational sac" can also appear in 5% of ectopic pregnancies.

A **yolk sac** appears between 6-7 weeks gestation on trans-abdominal pelvic ultrasound. The yolk sac is a thin-walled round structure about 1 cm in diameter located within the gestational sac. The presence of a yolk sac within a gestational sac is a definitive sign of an intra-uterine pregnancy.

A **fetal pole** appears between 7-8 weeks gestation on trans-abdominal pelvic ultrasound. The fetal pole appears as a hyperechoic (white) structure at the border of the yolk sac. The presence of a fetal pole is another definitive sign of an intra-uterine pregnancy.

Fetal cardiac activity can be observed between 7-8 weeks gestation on trans-abdominal pelvic ultrasound. The presence of intra-uterine fetal cardiac activity is diagnostic of a **live** intra-uterine pregnancy.

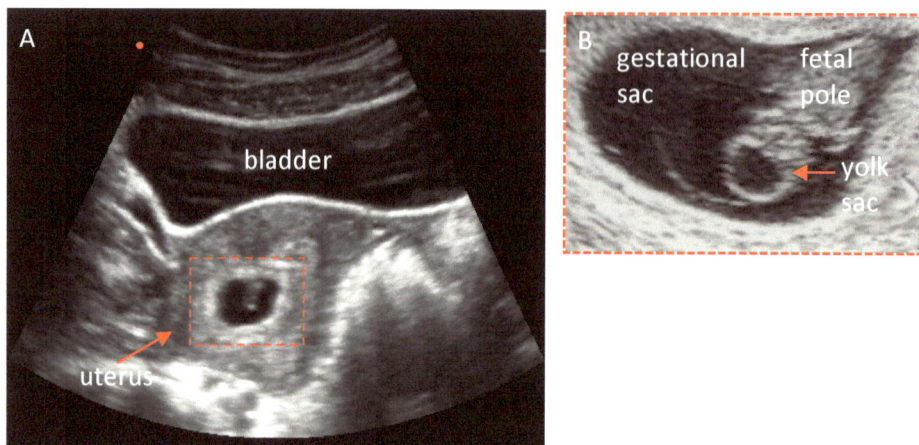

Figure 11.6 Gestational sac, yolk sac, and fetal pole imaged within the uterus in the transverse plane.

A. Female pelvis imaged in the transverse plane.
B. Enlarged view of the gestational sac, yolk sac, and fetal pole. Red circle denotes orientation marker.

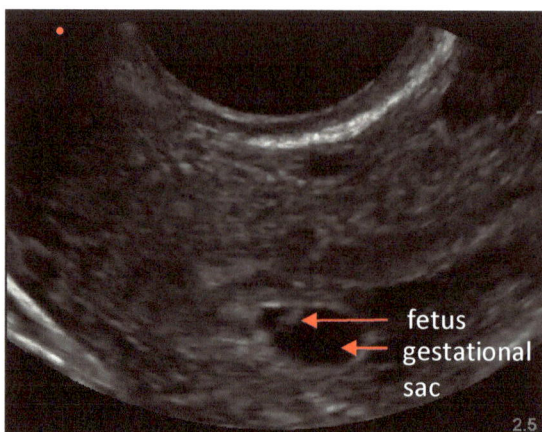

Video 11.1 Intra-uterine fetal cardiac activity on transvaginal ultrasound.

Red circle denotes orientation marker. View video online at bedsideultrasoundlevel1.com

11.4. Clinical relevance - Ectopic pregnancy

Ultrasound findings are used in combination with laboratory and clinical assessments in the management of suspected ectopic pregnancy.

In a patient suspected of having an ectopic pregnancy (Middleton, Kurtz et al., 2004; Nordenholz, Abbott et al., 2006; Reardon and Joing, 2008):

- The presence of an intra-uterine pregnancy excludes an ectopic pregnancy in the vast majority of cases. The exception to this rule is the heterotopic pregnancy (1:4000-8000 normal pregnancies; 1:100 pregnancies with assisted-reproductive techniques) where both intra-uterine and extra-uterine pregnancies occur simultaneously.

- The absence of an intra-uterine pregnancy suggests an ectopic pregnancy, particularly after 6 weeks of gestational age.

- Unstable vital signs, the absence of an intra-uterine pregnancy, and the presence of free pelvic or intraabdominal fluid (Chapter 6) is compelling evidence for a ruptured ectopic pregnancy.

11.5. Troubleshooting tips

- To improve the quality of pelvic ultrasound images, ensure that the patient's bladder is full.

- The uterus is generally imaged at a depth of 10-15 cm.

- When the uterus is not at the midline, its position is best determined by scanning in the transverse plane.

- If the gestational age is later than expected, the pregnant uterus may have entered the abdominal cavity.

Case closed:

The 30 year-old pregnant woman has no intra-uterine pregnancy identified on ultrasound examination. An ectopic pregnancy is suspected. She is transferred for urgent obstetrics consultation.

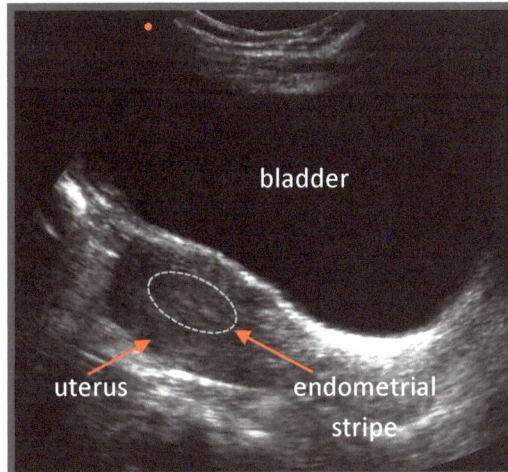

A normal female uterus imaged in the sagittal plane.

Index

Index

References

Amico, A. F., G. S. Lichtenberg, S. A. Reisner, C. K. Stone, R. G. Schwartz and R. S. Meltzer (1989). "Superiority of visual versus computerized echocardiographic estimation of radionuclide left ventricular ejection fraction." Am Heart J **118**(6): 1259-1265.

Anderson, B. (2000). Two-dimensional echocardiographic measurements and calculations. In Echocardiography: The normal examination and echocardiographic measurements. Brisbane, Australia, p 87-104.

Barnes, T. W., T. I. Morgenthaler, E. J. Olson, G. K. Hesley, P. A. Decker and J. H. Ryu (2005). "Sonographically guided thoracentesis and rate of pneumothorax." J Clin Ultrasound **33**(9): 442-446.

Birdwell, B. G., G. E. Raskob, T. L. Whitsett, S. S. Durica, P. C. Comp, J. N. George, T. L. Tytle and P. A. McKee (1998). "The clinical validity of normal compression ultrasonography in outpatients suspected of having deep venous thrombosis." Ann Intern Med **128**(1): 1-7.

Blaivas, M., M. J. Lambert, R. A. Harwood, J. P. Wood and J. Konicki (2000). "Lower-extremity Doppler for deep venous thrombosis--can emergency physicians be accurate and fast?" Acad Emerg Med **7**(2): 120-126.

Bree, R. L. (1995). "Further observations on the usefulness of the sonographic Murphy sign in the evaluation of suspected acute cholecystitis." J Clin Ultrasound **23**(3): 169-172.

Byrne, M., H. Kimberly and V. E. Noble (2013). Emergency renal ultrasonography. In Emergency medicine: Clinical essentials. J. G. Adams, E. D. Barton, J. Collings, P. M. C. DeBlieux, M. A. Gisondi and E. S. MNadel, eds, Saunders, p 998-1002.

Chan, H. (1993). "Noninvasive bladder volume measurement." J Neurosci Nurs **25**(5): 309-312.

Engel, J. M., E. A. Deitch and W. Sikkema (1980). "Gallbladder wall thickness: sonographic accuracy and relation to disease." AJR Am J Roentgenol **134**(5): 907-909.

Finberg, H. J. and J. C. Birnholz (1979). "Ultrasound evaluation of the gallbladder wall." Radiology **133**(3 Pt 1): 693-698.

Jackson, R. E., R. R. Rudoni, A. M. Hauser, R. G. Pascual and M. E. Hussey (2000). "Prospective evaluation of two-dimensional transthoracic echocardiography in emergency department patients with suspected pulmonary embolism." Acad Emerg Med **7**(9): 994-998.

Jardin, F., O. Dubourg and J. P. Bourdarias (1997). "Echocardiographic pattern of acute cor pulmonale." Chest **111**(1): 209-217.

Jones, P. W., J. P. Moyers, J. T. Rogers, R. M. Rodriguez, Y. C. Lee and R. W. Light (2003). "Ultrasound-guided thoracentesis: is it a safer method?" Chest **123**(2): 418-423.

Kelly, C. E. (2004). "Evaluation of voiding dysfunction and measurement of bladder volume." Rev Urol **6 Suppl 1**: S32-37.

Kircher, B. J., R. B. Himelman and N. B. Schiller (1990). "Noninvasive estimation of right atrial pressure from the inspiratory collapse of the inferior vena cava." Am J Cardiol **66**(4): 493-496.

Kirkpatrick, A. W., M. Sirois, K. B. Laupland, D. Liu, K. Rowan, C. G. Ball, S. M. Hameed, R. Brown, R. Simons, S. A. Dulchavsky, D. R. Hamiilton and S. Nicolaou (2004). "Hand-held thoracic sonography for detecting post-traumatic pneumothoraces: the Extended Focused Assessment with Sonography for Trauma (EFAST)." J Trauma 57(2): 288-295.

Labropoulos, N. and A. K. Tassiopoulos (2005). Vascular diagnosis of venous thrombosis. In Vascular diagnosis. M. A. Mansour and N. Labropoulos, eds. Philadelphia, Elsevier Saunders, p 429-438.

Lichtenstein, D. (2010). Introduction to lung ultrasound. In Whole body ultrasonography in the critically ill. Berlin Heidelberg, Springer, p 117-127.

Lichtenstein, D. and G. Meziere (1998). "A lung ultrasound sign allowing bedside distinction between pulmonary edema and COPD: the comet-tail artifact." Intensive Care Med 24(12): 1331-1334.

Lichtenstein, D., G. Meziere, P. Biderman and A. Gepner (2000). "The "lung point": an ultrasound sign specific to pneumothorax." Intensive Care Med 26(10): 1434-1440.

Lichtenstein, D. A. (2010). Pneumothorax. in Whole body ultrasonography in the critically ill. Berlin Heidelberg, Springer, p 163-179.

Lichtenstein, D. A. and Y. Menu (1995). "A bedside ultrasound sign ruling out pneumothorax in the critically ill. Lung sliding." Chest 108(5): 1345-1348.

Lichtenstein, D. A., G. Meziere, N. Lascols, P. Biderman, J. P. Courret, A. Gepner, I. Goldstein and M. Tenoudji-Cohen (2005). "Ultrasound diagnosis of occult pneumothorax." Crit Care Med 33(6): 1231-1238.

Lichtenstein, D. A. and G. A. Meziere (2008). "Relevance of lung ultrasound in the diagnosis of acute respiratory failure: the BLUE protocol." Chest 134(1): 117-125.

Lyon, M., M. Blaivas and L. Brannam (2005). "Sonographic measurement of the inferior vena cava as a marker of blood loss." Am J Emerg Med **23**(1): 45-50.

Ma, O. and J. Mateer (2008). Trauma. In Emergency Ultrasound. O. J. Ma, J. R. Mateer and M. Blaivas, eds. USA, McGraw Hill, p 77-108.

Magazzini, S., S. Vanni, S. Toccafondi, B. Paladini, M. Zanobetti, G. Giannazzo, R. Federico and S. Grifoni (2007). "Duplex ultrasound in the emergency department for the diagnostic management of clinically suspected deep vein thrombosis." Acad Emerg Med **14**(3): 216-220.

Middleton, W. D., A. B. Kurtz and B. S. Hertzberg (2004). The first trimester and ectopic pregnancy. in Ultrasound: The Requisites. St-Louis, MI, Mosby, p 342-373.

Middleton, W. D., A. B. Kurtz and B. S. Hertzberg (2004). General abdomen. in Ultrasound: The Requisites. St-Louis, MI, Mosby, p 220-243.

Mrabet, Y. (2012). "Human_anatomy_planes.svg." Wikimedia Commons.

Mueller, X., J. C. Stauffer, A. Jaussi, J. J. Goy and L. Kappenberger (1991). "Subjective visual echocardiographic estimate of left ventricular ejection fraction as an alternative to conventional echocardiographic methods: comparison with contrast angiography." Clin Cardiol **14**(11): 898-902.

Natori, H., S. Tamaki and S. Kira (1979). "Ultrasonographic evaluation of ventilatory effect on inferior vena caval configuration." Am Rev Respir Dis **120**(2): 421-427.

Noble, V. E., B. Nelson and A. N. Sutingco (2007). Abdominal aortic aneurysm. In Manual of emergency and critical care ultrasound. New York, Cambridge University Press, p 105-118.

Noble, V. E., B. Nelson and A. N. Sutingco (2007). First trimester ultrasound. In Manual of emergency and critical care ultrasound. New York, Cambridge University Press, p 85-103.

Noble, V. E., B. Nelson and A. N. Sutingco (2007). Focused asessment with sonography in Trauma (FAST). In Manual of emergency and critical care ultrasound. New York, Cambridge University Press, p 23-51.

Nordenholz, K., J. Abbott and J. Bailitz (2006). First trimester pregnancy. In Practical guide to emergency ultrasound. K. S. Cosby and J. L. Kendall, eds. Philadelphia, Lippincott Williams & Wilkins, p 124-160.

Ommen, S. R., R. A. Nishimura, D. G. Hurrell and K. W. Klarich (2000). "Assessment of right atrial pressure with 2-dimensional and Doppler echocardiography: a simultaneous catheterization and echocardiographic study." Mayo Clin Proc 75(1): 24-29.

Ouellet, J. F., C. G. Ball, N. L. Panebianco and A. W. Kirkpatrick (2011). "The sonographic diagnosis of pneumothorax." J Emerg Trauma Shock 4(4): 504-507.

Piette, E., R. Daoust and A. Denault (2013). "Basic concepts in the use of thoracic and lung ultrasound." Curr Opin Anaesthesiol 26(1): 20-30.

Poppiti, R., G. Papanicolaou, S. Perese and F. A. Weaver (1995). "Limited B-mode venous imaging versus complete color-flow duplex venous scanning for detection of proximal deep venous thrombosis." J Vasc Surg 22(5): 553-557.

Ralls, P. W., P. M. Colletti, S. A. Lapin, P. Chandrasoma, W. D. Boswell, Jr., C. Ngo, D. R. Radin and J. M. Halls (1985). "Real-time sonography in suspected acute cholecystitis. Prospective evaluation of primary and secondary signs." Radiology 155(3): 767-771.

Ralls, P. W., J. Halls, S. A. Lapin, M. F. Quinn, U. L. Morris and W. Boswell (1982). "Prospective evaluation of the sonographic Murphy sign in suspected acute cholecystitis." J Clin Ultrasound 10(3): 113-115.

Randazzo, M. R., E. R. Snoey, M. A. Levitt and K. Binder (2003). "Accuracy of emergency physician assessment of left ventricular ejection fraction and central venous pressure using echocardiography." Acad Emerg Med 10(9): 973-977.

Reardon, R. F., T. Cook and D. Plummer (2008). Abdominal aortic aneurysm. in Emergency Ultrasound. O. J. Ma, J. R. Mateer and M. Blaivas, eds. USA, McGraw Hill, p 149-167.

Reardon, R. F. and S. A. Joing (2008). Cardiac. In Emergency Ultrasound. O. J. Ma, J. R. Mateer and M. Blaivas, eds. USA, McGraw Hill, p 110-148.

Reardon, R. F. and S. A. Joing (2008). Frist trimester pregnancy. In Emergency Ultrasound. O. J. Ma, J. R. Mateer and M. Blaivas, eds. USA, McGraw Hill, p 179-318.

Shuman, W. P., W. Hastrup, Jr., T. R. Kohler, D. A. Nyberg, K. Y. Wang, L. M. Vincent and L. A. Mack (1988). "Suspected leaking abdominal aortic aneurysm: use of sonography in the emergency room." Radiology 168(1): 117-119.

Simonson, J. S. and N. B. Schiller (1988). "Sonospirometry: a new method for noninvasive estimation of mean right atrial pressure based on two-dimensional echographic measurements of the inferior vena cava during measured inspiration." J Am Coll Cardiol 11(3): 557-564.

Stamm, R. B., B. A. Carabello, D. L. Mayers and R. P. Martin (1982). "Two-dimensional echocardiographic measurement of left ventricular ejection fraction: prospective analysis of what constitutes an adequate determination." Am Heart J 104(1): 136-144.

Swadron, S. and D. Mandavia (2008). Renal. In Emergency Ultrasound. O. J. Ma, J. R. Mateer and M. Blaivas, eds. USA, McGraw Hill, p 230-255.

Tayal, V. S., C. D. Graf and M. A. Gibbs (2003). "Prospective study of accuracy and outcome of emergency ultrasound for abdominal aortic aneurysm over two years." Acad Emerg Med **10**(8): 867-871.

Tayal, V. S. and J. L. Kendall (2006). Trauma. In Practical guide to emergency ultrasound. K. S. Cosby and J. L. Kendall, eds. Philadelphia, Lippincott Williams & Wilkins, p 43-92.

Theodoro, D., M. Blaivas, S. Duggal, G. Snyder and M. Lucas (2004). "Real-time B-mode ultrasound in the ED saves time in the diagnosis of deep vein thrombosis (DVT)." Am J Emerg Med **22**(3): 197-200.

Wong, S. P. (2002). Echocardiographic findings in acute and chronic pulmonary disease. in The practice of clinical echocardiography. C. M. Otto, ed. Philadelphia, W.B. Saunders Company, p 739-760.

Yang, P. C., K. T. Luh, D. B. Chang, H. D. Wu, C. J. Yu and S. H. Kuo (1992). "Value of sonography in determining the nature of pleural effusion: analysis of 320 cases." AJR Am J Roentgenol **159**(1): 29-33.

Notes

CPSIA information can be obtained
at www.ICGtesting.com
Printed in the USA
BVHW02n0023270818
525651BV00013B/64/P